MW00625192

Primer of Palliative Care

6th Edition

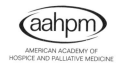

AMERICAN ACADEMY OF
HOSPICE AND PALLIATIVE MEDICINE

Primer of Palliative Care
6th Edition

Timothy E. Quill, MD FACP FAAHPM

Kimberly A. Bower, MD

Robert G. Holloway, MD MPH

Mindy Stevens Shah, MD

Thomas V. Caprio, MD MPH CMD FACP

Aaron Olden, MD MS

C. Porter Storey Jr., MD FACP FAAHPM

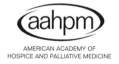

AMERICAN ACADEMY OF
HOSPICE AND PALLIATIVE MEDICINE

American Academy of Hospice and Palliative Medicine
8735 W. Higgins Road, Suite 300
Chicago, IL 60631
aahpm.org | PalliativeDoctors.org

The information presented and opinions expressed herein are those of the authors and do not necessarily represent the views of the American Academy of Hospice and Palliative Medicine. Any recommendations made by the authors must be weighed against the healthcare provider's own clinical judgment, based on but not limited to such factors as the patient's condition, benefits versus risks of suggested treatment, and comparison with recommendations of pharmaceutical compendia and other medical and palliative care authorities. Published in the United States by the American Academy of Hospice and Palliative Medicine, 8735 W. Higgins Road, Suite 300, Chicago, IL 60631.

© 2014 American Academy of Hospice and Palliative Medicine
First edition published 1994
Second edition published 1996
Third edition published 2004
Fourth edition published 2007
Fifth edition published 2010

ISBN 978-1-889296-13-5

Reviews of the *Primer* (Fifth Edition)

"The Primer *is an excellent resource for both the initiate and the seasoned professional. I tell our students and nurses that everything they need to know about hospice and palliative medicine is concisely and expertly described in the* Primer."

—Laurence Durante, MD MPH FAAHPM, St. Joseph Hospice & Palliative Care

"We use the Primer *as a core text for our nurses, nurse practitioners, and physicians. We highly recommend the* Primer *as a teaching tool and shared resource for patient care."*

—Geoff Galbraith, MD, Hospice Hawaii

"I order multiple copies of the Primer *to give to the medical school residents who come through our organization to learn more about end-of-life and hospice care. The* Primer *is a compendium of very valuable information for anyone caring for persons at the end of life, and especially those working in hospice and palliative care settings."*

—Morris Hoffpauir, MD, Hospice of Acadiana, Inc.

Foreword

The American Academy of Hospice and Palliative Medicine has just concluded a year of celebrations for its 25th anniversary, nearly 50 years after Cecily Saunders founded Saint Christopher's Hospice in South London. During the past quarter century, the number of hospice programs in the United States has grown to more than 5,500, and palliative care consultation services have become widely available in hospitals and clinics.

This edition of the *Primer* required considerable revision. The database in both hospice and hospital palliative care domains is growing rapidly, and much more evidence now exists to guide our practice. There will never be enough specialists in hospice and palliative medicine to care for all patients with advanced disease, and it is becoming apparent that primary palliative care knowledge and skills are essential for all who treat sick people. Recognizing that patients of all ages have palliative care needs, this edition includes a new pediatric palliative care chapter, skillfully written by Kimberly Bower, MD.

The coauthors and I are indebted to Tim Quill, MD FACP FAAHPM, for his excellent guidance and contributions to this edition. We are grateful to our mentors, especially Cecily Saunders and Balfour Mount (who kindly proofread the first edition of the *Primer*), and the courageous patients and heroic families who continue to inspire this important work. Although much has changed, patients with advanced disease still suffer from severe physical, psychological, financial, and spiritual distress and their care remains challenging—as Dr. Saunders reminded us:

> The work will at times cause pain and bewilderment to all members of the staff. If they do not have the opportunity of sharing their strain and questions, they are likely to leave this field or find a method of hiding behind a professional mask. Those who commit themselves to remaining near the suffering of dependence and parting find they are impelled to develop a basic philosophy, part individual and part corporate. This grows out of the work undertaken together as members find they have to search, often

painfully, for some meaning in the most adverse circumstances and gain enough freedom from their own anxieties to listen to another's questions of distress…

This search for meaning can create a climate in which patients and families can reach out in trust towards what they see as true and find acceptance of what is happening to them. We can, in some way, reach back into the ways of coming to terms with death of the past. The values the hospice movement tries to establish, alongside its commitment to excellence in practice, have something akin to the earlier assurance of community, the affirmation of the individual person, and the concern for the bereaved family (Saunders C. On dying well. Cambridge Review. 1984;24:49-54.).

C. Porter Storey Jr., MD FACP FAAHPM
Executive Vice President
American Academy of Hospice and Palliative Medicine

Preface

The sixth edition of the *Primer of Palliative Care* has been updated and expanded substantially from previous iterations. The biggest change is an entirely new chapter, Special Considerations for Infants and Children, authored by Kimberly Bower, MD, medical director of the pediatric program at Scripps Hospice. In addition to adult dosing recommendations, our enclosed equianalgesic pullout card now has weight- and age-based dosing recommendations for children, and the new pediatric chapter provides important recommendations for the palliative treatment of children in each of the domains from the first nine chapters. We also restructured chapter 5 (Delirium, Depression and Anxiety, Fatigue) and chapter 6 (Spiritual and Existential Suffering, the Search for Meaning, and Provider Self-Care) in this edition. Instead of offering a separate workbook, questions are included at the end of each chapter, which can be used to guide discussion among those using the book as a basic curriculum for palliative care training rotations. At the University of Rochester Medical Center, we provide a copy of the *Primer* to all trainees who do a palliative care rotation with us and use the discussion questions as a core part of their training curriculum.

All chapters have been updated and revised based on an extensive literature review. We screened each domain for new evidence-based information published over the past 4 years by searching the Cochrane Database, *PC-FACS*, *Clinical Practice Guidelines for Quality Palliative Care* (HPNA, 2013), *Evidence-Based Palliative Medicine* (Saunders, 2013), and by doing our own literature review for any new evidence-based studies. Although not a true systematic review, we made every effort to include evidence as it has emerged in hospice and palliative care since the *Primer* was last published in 2010. References for key articles used to update each domain are included at the end of each chapter, along with core articles from previous editions that still represent the state of the art and science, resulting in a net increase of about 100 articles for potential use by those seeking more in-depth exploration of a particular clinical question.

The goal for this book is to provide a basic resource to address common palliative care problems encountered by all clinicians who treat seriously ill patients, including primary care clinicians and specialists in virtually all fields, including palliative care. The treatment recommendations in this book allow clinicians at all levels to double check recommended palliative treatments, including specific starting doses for different populations and medications, and to search for commonly accepted alternative approaches. Palliative care specialists will sometimes require more information than is available herein to address the most challenging cases, but the information in this book will help all clinicians, both specialists and generalists, address the majority of common palliative care dilemmas that they will face in clinical practice. We hope you carry the book and the enclosed pain card with you, and use them regularly to help systematically address your patients' palliative care needs.

Acknowledgments

We are most grateful to the outstanding editorial staff at the American Academy of Hospice and Palliative Medicine (AAHPM) who have worked tirelessly to guide and support the chapter authors during this revision. Katie Macaluso was the chief editor and project coordinator, supported by senior managing editor Jerrod Liveoak, copyeditors Danielle Desjardins and Kelly Kellermann, graphic designers Terri Taylor and Amanda Monarch, director of education Julie Bruno, and education manager Kemi Ani, with additional guidance from Laura Davis, Jen Bose, Terrie McKissack, and Steve Smith. What a great group to work with!

We would like to thank Tamara Vesel, MD FAAHPM, for providing an external review of our new pediatric chapter. We recognize Kate Juba, PharmD, palliative care pharmacist at the University of Rochester Medical Center, for carefully reviewing our adult medication recommendations, and her colleague, David Hutchinson, PharmD, for providing a similar pharmaceutical review for the pediatric section. The external reviewers of the fifth edition of the *Primer* and AAHPM Clinical Education Committee members Rebekah Halpern, MS PA-C; Scott Schwantes, MD; and Denise Waugh, MD FAAHPM, helped guide us at the beginning of this revision.

As always, we remain grateful to the many patients, families, and staff members with whom we have had the privilege of working in hospice and palliative care over the years, who provide such a meaningful subtext for the information contained in this book.

Authors

Timothy E. Quill, MD FACP FAAHPM
Gosnell Distinguished Professor in Palliative Care
Director, Palliative Care Program
University of Rochester Medical Center
Rochester, NY

Kimberly A. Bower, MD
Medical Director, Pediatric Program
Scripps Hospice
San Diego, CA

Robert G. Holloway, MD MPH
Professor of Neurology and Public Health Sciences
Chair, Department of Neurology
University of Rochester Medical Center
Rochester, NY

Mindy Stevens Shah, MD
Assistant Professor of Clinical Medicine
Associate Medical Director, Visiting Nurse Hospice and Palliative Care
University of Rochester Medical Center
Rochester, NY

Thomas V. Caprio, MD MPH CMD FACP
Assistant Professor of Medicine, Clinical Nursing, and Public Health
Sciences
Director, Geriatric Medicine Fellowship Program
Medical Director, Visiting Nurse Hospice and Palliative Care
University of Rochester Medical Center
Rochester, NY

Aaron Olden, MD MS
Clinical Instructor of Medicine
University of Rochester Medical Center
Rochester, NY

C. Porter Storey Jr., MD FACP FAAHPM
Executive Vice President
American Academy of Hospice and Palliative Medicine
Colorado Permanente Medical Group
Boulder, CO

Contents

Tables

Figures

ONE

Introduction

Patients with advanced disease need and deserve excellent symptom management; capable psychosocial support; assistance with difficult medical decision making; and warm, healing relationships with their professional caregivers. Palliative care is a field developed to help meet these needs for patients and their families. Palliative care is potentially appropriate for patients at all stages of serious illness, whereas hospice is a specialized form of palliative care for patients who are in the terminal stages of illness.[1]

All clinicians who care for seriously ill patients should have the skills to provide basic palliative care. The purpose of this introductory guide is to assist you in providing basic palliative care to all patients with advanced disease, to offer tools to address common palliative care dilemmas, and to provide resources to help improve your skills. For more complex palliative care problems, or for patients who do not respond to basic interventions, specialist-level palliative care consultations should be seriously considered.[2]

In the first nine chapters, comments and recommendations will be restricted to adults. In the newly added chapter 10, additional special considerations and helpful references and resources for delivering basic palliative care to children will be discussed.

1A | Definitions

The *Clinical Practice Guidelines for Quality Palliative Care*, developed as part of the National Consensus Project (NCP), defines *palliative care* as follows[3]:

> *Palliative care means patient- and family-centered care that optimizes quality of life by anticipating, preventing, and treating suffering. Palliative care throughout the continuum of illness involves addressing physical, intellectual, emotional, social, and*

spiritual needs to facilitate patient autonomy, access to information, and choice.

The following features characterize palliative care philosophy and delivery:

- *Care is provided and services are coordinated by an interdisciplinary team.*
- *Patients, families, and palliative and non-palliative healthcare providers collaborate and communicate about care needs.*
- *Services are available concurrently with or independent of curative or life-prolonging care.*
- *Patient and family hopes for peace and dignity are supported throughout the course of illness, during the dying process, and at death.*

Prior versions of the NCP specifically describe palliative care delivery as follows: Palliative care is operationalized through effective management of pain and other distressing symptoms, while incorporating psychosocial and spiritual care with consideration of patient/family needs, preferences, values, beliefs, and culture. Evaluation and treatment should be comprehensive and patient-centered, with a focus on the central role of the family unit in decision making. Palliative care affirms life by supporting the patient's and family's goals for the future, including their hopes for cure or life prolongation, as well as their hopes for peace and dignity throughout the course of illness, including the dying process and death.

The effort to integrate palliative care into all health care for persons with debilitating, potentially life-threatening illnesses is designed to ensure that the following objectives are met:

- Pain and symptom control, psychosocial distress, spiritual issues, and practical needs are addressed with the patient and family throughout the continuum of care.
- Patients and families obtain the information they need to fully understand the illness, prognosis, and treatment options. During this

process, the goals of patients and families are elicited, the benefits and burdens of treatment are regularly reassessed, and decision making about treatment is sensitive to changes in the patient's condition. If there is conflict among the patient, the family, and the treatment team, palliative care providers sometimes take a leadership role in approaching and resolving these often complex situations.

- Genuine coordination of care across settings is ensured through regular, high-quality communication between providers at times of transition or changing needs and through effective continuity of care using case management techniques.
- If death is anticipated, the patient and family are given the opportunity to prepare, including exploring the option for hospice care. Opportunities for personal growth are maximized, and bereavement support is made available for the family.

The National Hospice and Palliative Care Organization defines *hospice* as follows[4]:

> Considered to be the model for quality, compassionate care for people facing a life-limiting illness or injury, hospice and palliative care involve a team-oriented approach to expert medical care, pain management, and emotional and spiritual support expressly tailored to the person's needs and wishes. Support is provided to the person's loved ones as well.
>
> The focus of hospice relies on the belief that each of us has the right to die pain free and with dignity, and that our loved ones will receive the necessary support to allow us to do so.

- *Hospice focuses on caring, not curing, and in most cases, care is provided in the person's home.*
- *Hospice care also is provided in freestanding hospice centers, hospitals, and nursing homes and other long-term care facilities.*
- *Hospice services are available to patients of any age, religion, race, or illness.*
- *Hospice care is covered under Medicare, Medicaid, most private insurance plans, HMOs, and other managed care organizations.*

1B | Illness Trajectories and Palliative Care

The four trajectories of functional decline before dying have implications for palliative care and healthcare delivery (**Figure 1.1**).[5] Patients and families have different physical, psychological, social, and spiritual needs, depending on the likely trajectory of their illness before they die. Awareness of these trajectories can help providers anticipate and deliver appropriate care that integrates both disease-directed and palliative treatments.

Trajectory 1: Short period of evident decline before death. Cancer typifies this trajectory. Function is generally preserved until late in the disease course, followed by a predictable and precipitous decline over weeks to months. The onset of decline usually suggests worsening metastatic disease. A predictable decline in function allows for more accurate prognoses and can assist in anticipating care needs. This functional decline may facilitate the transition from disease-directed treatments toward a more exclusive emphasis on palliation and eventually hospice care. Not all malignancies follow this trajectory (eg, prostate or breast cancer), and some nonmalignant conditions may also follow this course (eg, amyotrophic lateral sclerosis).

Trajectory 2: Chronic illness with exacerbations and sudden dying. Congestive heart failure, chronic obstructive pulmonary disease, end-stage liver disease, and AIDS typify this trajectory. These organ-system diseases represent chronic illnesses with high symptom burdens and increasing care needs. The course of illness is characterized by periodic, acute exacerbations (eg, physiological stress that overwhelms the body's reserves) that require increased levels of care (eg, hospital admission). Patients can improve functionally after an exacerbation, but often do not return to their prior baseline. Prognosticating is very challenging because these patients are at risk for sudden death but may stabilize for prolonged periods. When patients choose to forgo or stop aggressive, life-sustaining therapies, planning for aggressive symptom relief during a future exacerbation is essential.

Trajectory 3: Progressive deterioration. Neurodegenerative disease (eg, dementia, Parkinson's disease, advanced multiple sclerosis) and frailty

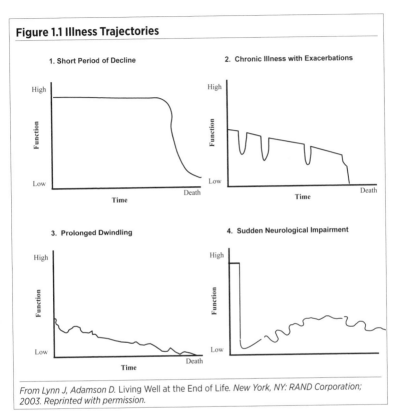

Figure 1.1 Illness Trajectories

1. Short Period of Decline

Function (High to Low) vs Time (to Death)

2. Chronic Illness with Exacerbations

Function (High to Low) vs Time (to Death)

3. Prolonged Dwindling

Function (High to Low) vs Time (to Death)

4. Sudden Neurological Impairment

Function (High to Low) vs Time

From Lynn J, Adamson D. Living Well at the End of Life. *New York, NY: RAND Corporation; 2003. Reprinted with permission.*

typify this trajectory. These patients have a prolonged course of gradual physical and cognitive decline with increasing fatigue, weight loss, and declining oral intake. Multiple comorbidities, including arthritis, loss of vision, prior stroke, heart disease, and diabetes contribute to declining physiological reserve and function. Caregiver support is challenging and crucial if the patient is to remain at home. Prognosticating survival is difficult, and infectious complications (eg, pneumonia, urinary tract infections, decubiti) and fractures may be terminal events. The (relatively few) benefits and (many) burdens of artificial nutrition and hydration must often be addressed.

Trajectory 4: Sudden, severe neurological injury. Diagnoses that lead to sudden and often severe neurological impairment (ie, stroke, hypoxic ischemic encephalopathy, traumatic brain injury) typify this trajectory. Deaths can occur in the acute stages as a result of brain injury, from complications despite full treatment efforts, or after treatments are withheld or withdrawn. Familiarity with organ donation policies and procedures is essential. Prognosticating is challenging given the uncertainties in predicting neurological outcome as well as the time required to allow for optimal recovery (sometimes months). These injuries are the leading cause of adult disability. At the extremes of impairment are persistent vegetative states, minimally conscious states, and locked-in syndromes, but there is a vast spectrum of impairments short of these extremes. This trajectory requires a healthcare system prepared for and responsive to negotiating goals of treatment with patients and surrogates, and raises questions about how to manage patients with potentially severe physical and cognitive debility and varying chances of improvement.

1C | Introducing Palliative Care to Patients

Patients with serious, potentially life-threatening illnesses and their families are very vulnerable and initially may be frightened about the prospect of receiving palliative care (**Figure 1.2**). This fear primarily is because of the potential confusion between palliative care and end-of-life care.[6] Such concerns can be addressed by reinforcing to patients and families how palliative care augments their usual treatment plan. Palliative care

- helps address pain and other uncomfortable symptoms
- assists with understanding and making difficult medical decisions
- provides additional support for patients and families during a difficult illness
- usually is delivered alongside the best possible disease-directed treatments.

After understanding and addressing dimensions of potential suffering and getting to know patients and their families, palliative care consultants can help establish patient-centered goals of care, including

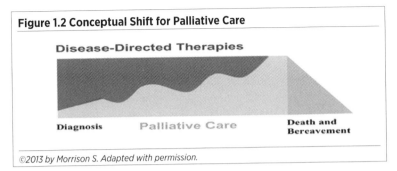

Figure 1.2 Conceptual Shift for Palliative Care

Disease-Directed Therapies

Diagnosis   Palliative Care   Death and Bereavement

advance care planning, the role of additional medical consultations, and residential options to best meet the patient's needs and goals. They can address patients' wishes with regard to cardiopulmonary resuscitation, intubation, and other potentially life-sustaining interventions (especially under circumstances that would indicate such treatments have a high burden and low likelihood of success). In such circumstances, the challenge is for patients and families to simultaneously

- hope for the best (explore all treatments that might help prolong life and relieve suffering, including traditional and experimental therapies)
- prepare for the worst (consider what would be left undone if treatment does not go as hoped; who should make decisions for the patient if decision-making capacity is lost in the future; and what, if any, limits might be set right now on aggressive treatments such as cardiopulmonary resuscitation).

Both clinicians and patients may find addressing these questions at the same time challenging, yet both are necessary to give the patient the best possible treatment, given his or her values and clinical circumstances.[7]

1D | Introducing Hospice to Patients

For most patients, referral to hospice means an increase in the intensity of home services. It also means an increase in the supportive resources available to them. Under the Medicare hospice benefit, costs of care related to palliating a terminal illness are covered without a deductible. This coverage benefit includes medications, some caregiver services, and supplies. Hospice usually can provide up to 2 to 4 hours of home health aide services each day, so families will need to be prepared and able to provide the majority of the "hands-on" care needed if a hospice patient stays at home. Hospice also can supplement care in a skilled nursing facility, but patients themselves or their insurance (generally Medicaid) would be responsible for the nursing home room and board charges. The hospice benefit also includes bereavement care (counseling and support) for the family after the patient's death. A referral to hospice does not mean the medical team will discontinue caring for the patient, nor will the medical team stop striving for the patient to live "as well as possible, for as long as possible."[8]

Some patients and families initially may experience the transition to hospice as a form of "giving up" on active treatment and "giving in" to death. These potential responses may need to be explored before those patients and families are able to understand and appreciate some of the opportunities for personal growth, psychosocial support, and transcendence that hospice potentially provides. The initial introduction of hospice, therefore, may require strategies and preparations similar to those used for delivering "bad news,"[9] including the ability to respond to strong emotion with care and compassion. This is particularly relevant when patients and families are being made aware of and appreciating for the first time that the burdens of treatments intended to prolong life now outweigh their benefits. In preparation for these discussions, the clinician should be fully informed about the benefits and burdens of the patient's remaining medical options and should discuss potential approaches with the patient's primary physician, medical specialists, and other providers (eg, nurses, therapists) to see whether there is a consensus about hospice being the best approach. This preparation may include gathering information about what the patient and family had previously been told, and how receptive they have been to discussions about treatment goals and limitations and hospice. For specific guidance about how to establish patient-centered goals and effectively run family meetings, see chapter 7.

1E | Teamwork

Work with seriously ill patients can be very emotionally and intellectually rewarding, but the intensity of the work and the exposure to human suffering and frailty can increase the risks of burnout and job dissatisfaction. One way that palliative care and hospice practitioners have learned to counteract this danger is to share the work and challenges as part of a multidisciplinary team, as well as to pay attention to personal strategies for self-care.[10,11] Clinicians who are not fortunate enough to work as a part of such teams would do well to develop a small group of trusted colleagues to regularly discuss and share the burden of caring for such critically ill patients and families over time.

Team meetings can become more interesting, educational, and productive for better patient care if you take three important steps:

1. **Develop genuine collegial relationships with other professionals and volunteers.** Listen carefully and learn from each other. The real test of your success at becoming a team member is whether your colleagues feel comfortable challenging as well as supporting you.

2. **Genuinely learn to respect and appreciate the views and opinions of others.** Becoming an effective team member is to recognize that each member contributes uniquely to the work and to respect the views of those with different areas of expertise. Team functioning and personal well-being are greatly enhanced by building and practicing team-based skills. Your efforts will improve the quality of your patients' care, your relationships with your colleagues, and your own job satisfaction.

3. **Take care of yourself.**[10,11] Treating and caring for patients and families with advanced illness, many of whom die, can lead to stress, job dissatisfaction, or even professional burnout. Active steps to confront these risks are critical for effective professional and team behavior and function. For ways to address and approach these issues, see chapter 6.

Further Discussion

1. Name three key elements of palliative care.
2. Name three key elements of hospice.
3. Name three ways in which hospice is different from palliative care.
4. Name three clinical indications for discussing palliative care.
5. Name three clinical indications for discussing hospice.
6. Name two barriers to discussing palliative care.
7. Name two barriers to discussing hospice.
8. Does a patient need to have a do-not-resuscitate order to be accepted into a hospice program?
9. To qualify for hospice, how likely does it have to be that a patient will die in the next 6 months?

References

1. Morrison RS, Meier DE. Clinical practice. Palliative care. *N Engl J Med.* 2004;350(25):2582-2590.

2. Quill TE, Abernethy AP. Generalist plus specialist palliative care—creating a more sustainable model. *N Engl J Med.* 2013;368(13):1173-1175.

3. National Consensus Project for Quality Palliative Care. *Clinical Practice Guidelines for Quality Palliative Care*. 3rd ed. Pittsburgh, PA: National Consensus Project for Quality Palliative Care; 2013. www.national consensusproject.org/NCP_Clinical_Practice_Guidelines_3rd_Edition. pdf. Accessed October 8, 2013.

4. National Hospice and Palliative Care Organization. Hospice. www.caringinfo.org/i4a/pages/index.cfm?pageid=3356. Accessed October 8, 2013.

5. Murray SA, Kendall M, Boyd K, Sheikh A. Illness trajectories and palliative care. *BMJ.* 2005;330(7498):1007-1011.

6. Quill TE. Perspectives on care at the close of life. Initiating end-of-life discussions with seriously ill patients: addressing the "elephant in the room." *JAMA*. 2000;284(19):2502-2507.

7. Back AL, Arnold RM, Quill TE. Hope for the best, and prepare for the worst. *Ann Intern Med*. 2003;138(5):439-443.

8. von Gunten CF. Discussing hospice care. *J Clin Oncol*. 2002;20(5):1419-1424.

9. Casarett DJ, Quill TE. "I'm not ready for hospice": strategies for timely and effective hospice discussions. *Ann Intern Med*. 2007;146(6):443-449.

10. Quill TE, Williamson PR. Healthy approaches to physician stress. *Arch Intern Med*. 1990;150:1857-1861.

11. Meier DE, Back AL, Morrison RS. The inner life of physicians and care of the seriously ill. *JAMA*. 2001;286(23):3007-3014.

·

TWO

Pain Management

Most pain can be brought under adequate control, if not completely eliminated, with the diligent application of basic pain management principles that should be part of the knowledge and skill sets of all clinicians who care for patients with serious illness. Experts in pain management and palliative care should be consulted when basic pain management strategies are insufficient. A careful patient history, screen for addiction risk factors, caregiver or family interview, record review, physical examination, and a look at available laboratory data and imaging studies are essential.

Attempts should be made to characterize the quality of the pain as somatic (eg, constant, localized, changing with movement), visceral (eg, deep, aching, cramping, poorly localized), or neuropathic (eg, burning, shooting, tingling, shock-like). The intensity of the pain should be measured on a 0 (*no pain*) to 10 (*extremely severe pain*) scale, and this intensity should be repeatedly quantified over time to assess treatment efficacy. In nonverbal or cognitively impaired patients, listen to caregivers, watch the patient's facial expressions and body language, and carefully observe the effects of trial dosages of analgesics. **Figure 2.1** shows representative pain scales for verbal and nonverbal patients. Although the goal in terms of targeted pain intensity level should be negotiated with the individual patient, moderate pain levels (4 to 6 on a 10-point scale) generally interfere with function and sleep, and severe pain levels (7/10 to 10/10) additionally interfere with concentration. Mild levels of pain (lower than 4/10) usually can be kept in the background, allowing for more normal function and engagement. Always remember that psychological, social, spiritual, or financial problems can affect a patient's perception and tolerance of pain.

This chapter focuses primarily on treating pain with opioid analgesics. It also presents a brief overview of adjuvant analgesics and invasive treatment options. Methadone and fentanyl are broken out in section 2B from the more general section describing opioid conversions (section 2A) because of some special considerations in dosage transitioning. The treatment of pain also should involve a multidimensional approach that includes the optimization of nonpharmacologic treatments and requests for additional consults (eg, pain specialists, addiction specialists, radiation oncologists, mental health professionals, neurosurgeons, complementary medicine experts) as needed.

Figure 2.1 Scales for Measuring Pain Intensity

Numeric Pain Rating Scale

Rate your pain on a scale of 0 (*no pain*) to 10 (*extremely severe pain*).

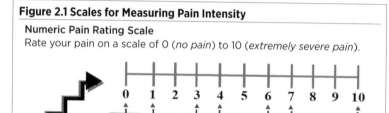

Pain Assessment in Advanced Dementia (PAINAD) Scale

Items*	0	1	2	Score
Breathing independent of vocalization	Normal	Occasional labored breathing. Short period of hyperventilation.	Noisy labored breathing. Long period of hyperventilation. Cheyne-Stokes respirations.	
Negative vocalization	None	Occasional moan or groan. Low-level speech with a negative or disapproving quality.	Repeated troubled calling out. Loud moaning or groaning. Crying.	
Facial expression	Smiling or inexpressive	Sad. Frightened. Frown.	Facial grimacing.	
Body language	Relaxed	Tense. Distressed pacing. Fidgeting.	Rigid. Fists clenched. Knees pulled up. Pulling or pushing away. Striking out.	
Consolability	No need to console	Distracted or reassured by voice or touch.	Unable to console, distract or reassure.	
			Total**	

*Five-item observational tool.

**Total scores range from 0 to 10 (based on a scale of 0 to 2 for five items), with a higher score indicating more severe pain (0 = "no pain" to 10 = "severe pain").

From Walden V, Hurley AC, Volicer L. Development and psychometric evaluation of the pain assessment in advanced dementia (PAINAD) scale. J Am Med Dir Assoc. 2003;4(1):9-15.
© 2003 Elsevier. All rights reserved. Adapted with permission.

2A | Opioids

The skillful use of opioid analgesics may improve many types of acute and chronic pain. Although opioids are a cornerstone in the relief of chronic pain for patients who are terminally ill, their use in patients with chronic nonmalignant pain and those who have risk factors for opioid abuse remains much more challenging and controversial (see section 2E).[1] See the foldout Equianalgesic Table for Adults and Children (**Table 2.1**) for information and guidelines on opioid use.

Choosing an Analgesic

Mild pain may respond well to nonopioid analgesics such as acetaminophen or a nonsteroidal anti-inflammatory drug (NSAID). Mild to moderate pain often has been treated with combination products containing both acetaminophen and a weak opioid, although this practice has fallen out of favor because of the potential for acetaminophen toxicity. Moderate to severe pain generally should be treated with a strong opioid in the absence of significant risk factors for addiction and abuse. There are no strict rules to follow when choosing between strong opioids. For many patients, generic morphine is a reasonable initial choice because of its efficacy and relatively low cost. In specific situations, however, other agents may be preferable:

- **Renal insufficiency:** Hydromorphone or oxycodone can be used with caution, but may require dosage reductions or increasing dosing intervals if adverse effects develop. Avoid using morphine in cases of renal insufficiency because of the potential for accumulation of active metabolites.[2] Regarding pharmacokinetics, methadone and fentanyl appear to be optimal because of their inactive metabolites. Notably, methadone and fentanyl are likely the best agents for patients on dialysis because they are not dialyzed.[3] See section 2B regarding cautions about methadone and fentanyl prescribing.
- **Hepatic insufficiency:** Fentanyl, hydromorphone, oxycodone, and methadone can be used with caution. Again, dose reductions or increased dosing intervals may be required. Avoid morphine because of the potential accumulation of active metabolites.

- **Older adults:** Older adults may have reduced renal function, necessitating the use of analgesics with fewer active metabolites. However, opioids should not be withheld from older adults in pain.[4] Instead, reduce starting dosages, titrate gradually using small increments, and monitor for side effects, including changes in mental status or excessive sedation (see Table 2.1).
- **Cost:** Methadone may have significant cost advantages over other opioids, but its long and variable half-life makes it challenging to use for inexperienced providers (see below). Prescribers are strongly advised to use generics whenever possible. (Table 2.1 also has relative cost information.)

Designing an Opioid Regimen

Moderate and severe chronic pain should be treated with a combination of the following:

- **Scheduled "around the clock" dosing:** Most short-acting opioids last 3 to 4 hours; therefore, scheduled dosing should begin every 4 hours around the clock and be adjusted to every 3 hours if the analgesic effect fades in the last hour. Scheduled dosing is especially vital for patients with cognitive impairment or decreased mental status who may not be able to request as-needed (prn) medication. Once an effective total daily dosage of an opioid is determined (usually a stable total of scheduled doses and prn doses over 24 hours), the patient may be switched to a long-acting opioid for the scheduled dosing for ease of administration. The interval for prn dosing may be longer in older adults or those with renal or hepatic impairment. If it appears that the baseline dosage needs to be adjusted, keep in mind that it may take 2 to 3 days for an extended-release opioid (and 3 to 6 days for transdermal fentanyl) to reach a steady state, so daily changes in longer-acting medications are inadvisable in most situations.
- **As-needed doses for breakthrough pain:** In general, the prn dose should be approximately 10% of the total daily dose, given every 1 to 2 hours orally (PO) or every 30 to 60 minutes for subcutaneous (SC) or intravenous (IV) agents (recommended prn intervals are based on the average time from dose administration to peak effect). For

patients receiving a continuous infusion of opioids with the ability to use a patient-controlled analgesia (PCA) pump, another way to administer prn dosing is to give the basal rate hourly dose as a bolus every 15 minutes prn through the PCA pump. Frequent assessments of prn usage should be performed to determine if patients need a change in their scheduled medication; prn doses should not be relied upon for those in persistent pain. Prn dosing must be much more conservative in patients with risk factors for addiction, including limiting the total number of doses available in a 24-hour period and generally having them delivered by a nurse rather than a PCA pump.

For patients who can take PO medications, tablets or liquids are preferred because they are effective, convenient, oftentimes less expensive, and have fewer serious complications. Patients unable to take PO medications or those with significant absorption problems can use transdermal (TD), SC, or IV routes. In general, the least invasive route is preferable: from PO to TD to SC to IV. TD and SC routes may not be optimal if skin integrity is compromised or if the patient is severely cachectic. For some patients, rectal administration of medications may be feasible; however, it is prudent to check with a pharmacist regarding the reliability of absorption of the medication being considered.

When a patient needs to switch from one opioid to another, either because of tolerance or side effects, the calculated equianalgesic amount of the new opioid usually should be lowered by 30% to 50% because of incomplete cross-tolerance.[5,6] For patients with poorly controlled pain, such a reduction may be inappropriate because the unadjusted equianalgesic dose will equate with a 30% to 50% dose increase. Conversion ratios are listed in Table 2.1. Rotation from other opioids to methadone and fentanyl is an exception to this rule; see the section below on special considerations.

Sample Calculation 1. Conversion Between PO and IV Routes

(See Table 2.1 for equianalgesic doses and a summary of conversion guidelines.)

A 62-year-old man with metastatic colon cancer is taking 60 mg of sustained-release PO morphine twice daily, with 15-mg tablets of immediate-release PO morphine available every 2 hours prn. He is using four prn doses per day. His pain level is 5/10 (moderate), and he now has a partial bowel obstruction. Because of his moderately high pain level, you need to increase his baseline opioid dose. You also must change the route of administration while the cause of nausea and emesis is investigated and treated.

Step 1. Calculate the total daily dose.

The total daily dose of morphine is the total scheduled dose plus the total prn use as follows:

- 120 mg sustained-release PO morphine per day (two doses of 60 mg) + 60 mg immediate-release PO morphine per day (15 mg × four doses) = 180 mg PO morphine per day total.

Step 2. Convert to IV morphine.

The conversion ratio of PO morphine to IV morphine is 3:1 (see Table 2.1) as follows:

- 180 mg PO morphine × 1 mg IV morphine/3 mg PO morphine = 60 mg IV morphine.

Therefore, the patient will require a total of 60 mg IV morphine per day to achieve the same level of analgesia (equianalgesic total of prior baseline and prn doses that provided pain relief in the moderate zone, 5/10). (SC administration would be another possible route and would follow the same dose conversion guidelines.)

Step 3. Determine the scheduled dose.

Around-the-clock IV morphine can be given in intermittent doses every 4 hours or by continuous infusion as follows:

- If the morphine is given every 4 hours (based on its usual duration of analgesic activity), the patient will receive a total of six doses per day.

Divide the total daily dose of IV morphine into six doses: 60 mg IV morphine per day divided by six doses = 10 mg IV morphine every 4 hours around the clock.

- If a continuous infusion was ordered, then the 60 mg total IV morphine per day would be divided by 24 hours: 60 mg/24 hours = 2.5 mg IV morphine per hour by continuous infusion.

In general, the baseline infusion rate of an opioid should not be increased more often than every 12 hours unless the patient is in an acute pain crisis (see section 2C).

Step 4. Determine the prn dose.

- The prn dose usually should be 10% of the total daily dose given every 1 to 2 hours if oral or every 30 to 60 minutes if parenteral: 10% of 60 mg IV morphine = 6 mg IV morphine every 30 to 60 minutes prn.

If the patient is receiving a continuous baseline infusion, another way to order the prn dose is to repeat the hourly rate every 15 minutes prn using a PCA pump: 2.5 mg every 15 minutes prn.

The Case Continues

The patient's pain is well controlled on the IV morphine, needing only one prn dose at bedtime. The dose has been stable for several days. He has developed moderate renal insufficiency, so you decide to rotate him off of morphine because of concern about the accumulation of active metabolites. Because his partial bowel obstruction has resolved, you take advantage of the availability of the PO route and opt for oxycodone. You plan to convert him to short-acting oxycodone and hope to transition him to long-acting oxycodone once his pain has stabilized.

Step 5. Convert to immediate-release oxycodone.

As can be seen in Table 2.1, the conversion from IV morphine to PO oxycodone requires calculating an equianalgesic amount as follows:

- Total daily dosage of IV morphine is 60 mg IV morphine per day baseline + 6 mg prn doses per day = 66 mg IV morphine per day.

- Calculating an equianalgesic amount of PO oxycodone: The ratio of IV morphine to PO morphine is 1:3, so 66 mg IV morphine is equal to 198 mg PO morphine. The ratio of PO morphine to PO oxycodone is 3:2, so 198 mg oral morphine is equal to 132 mg of oral oxycodone. (Note. The equianalgesic card [Table 2.1] is fully integrated for morphine, oxycodone, and hydromorphone.) The ratio of IV morphine to PO oxycodone is 1:2, so 66 mg IV morphine per day could be converted directly to the equianalgesic equivalent of 132 mg PO oxycodone per day.
- Incomplete cross-tolerance should always be considered when changing opioids, so in a patient with well-controlled pain, the equianalgesic amount should be decreased by approximately one-third: 132 mg × ⅔ = 88 mg. (Note. For those with persistent moderate to severe pain, using the equianalgesic amount without the dose reduction for cross-tolerance potentially could achieve a 30% increase in effective analgesia).
- When immediate-release opioids are used as baseline treatment for chronic pain, they should be given every 3 to 4 hours based on their relatively short half-life. Therefore, the 88 mg total daily dosage of oxycodone could be divided into six doses of approximately 15 mg, to be given every 4 hours around the clock.

Step 6. Calculate the new prn medication and dose.
The prn dose should be the same medication class as the baseline medication whenever possible, and should be approximately 10% of the total daily dosage.

The patient will receive a total equivalent of about 90 mg PO oxycodone per day. Ten percent of this would be 9 mg, which could be rounded up to 10 mg per prn dose; this dose could be given every 1 to 2 hours prn for pain that was not adequately controlled by the baseline regimen.

The Case Continues
The patient's pain was able to be maintained in the mild range over the next several days with a combination of the baseline oxycodone of 15

mg every 4 hours around the clock and an average of three prn doses of 10 mg each. The patient is swallowing well and eager to not take medication so frequently. You decide to initiate a long-acting opioid for baseline pain control.

Step 7. Transition to long-acting medication as baseline, if possible.
- The first step in transitioning to a long-acting preparation is to calculate the total daily dosage. Taking 15 mg of oxycodone every 4 hours is 90 mg per day, plus three prn doses of 10 mg (30 additional mg), resulting in a total daily oxycodone dose of 120 mg.
- Long-acting oxycodone generally is given every 12 hours. In Table 2.1, the available dosage options of each medication are provided. Long-acting oxycodone comes in 60-mg tablets, so it could be given as 60 mg extended-release oxycodone every 12 hours as the baseline medication.
- The patient will still need an immediate-release medication for break-through pain. It should be 10% of the total daily dosage (10% of 120 mg = 12 mg, which could be rounded down to 10 mg per dose or rounded up to 15 mg); the interval of the prn dosing should be every 1 to 2 hours based on the time from ingestion to peak effect. Therefore the final dose would be 60 mg extended-release oxycodone every 12 hours and 10 mg immediate-release oxycodone every 1 hour prn for breakthrough pain.

2B | Fentanyl and Methadone
Special Considerations
Both fentanyl and methadone have been designated by expert panels as exceptions to the usual conversion rules for morphine, oxycodone, and hydromorphone. Clinicians planning to prescribe these medications must familiarize themselves with these distinct rules and ask for help from experienced providers if they are unsure about how to proceed or if they are converting large dosages.

Transdermal Fentanyl

The conversion ratios from PO morphine to TD fentanyl shown in Table 2.1 are based on tables created by the manufacturer that already included a correction factor for incomplete cross-tolerance, so the routine reduction of the equianalgesic amount by 30% to 50% is probably not necessary. However, because manufacturers' guidelines do not necessarily cover converting from fentanyl to another opioid, it may be wise to use the most conservative end of the range when converting away from fentanyl (ie, reduce the calculated equianalgesic amount by 50% rather than 30%). Patients should be carefully observed and prn doses made readily available during this transition in case the conversion is too conservative.

When administered transdermally, fentanyl absorption can be affected by tissue perfusion and skin integrity. Absorption can be increased by an elevated body temperature, making TD fentanyl occasionally problematic in febrile patients. TD fentanyl is stored in adipose tissue and then gradually released. This means it takes 12 to 24 hours to take full effect, and it will take 12 to 24 hours to be eliminated once the patch is removed. This stable, slow release makes it easy to manage once a steady state is achieved (usually it will last 72 hours between changing patches), but it is very difficult to use in situations where pain levels or the patient's clinical condition change rapidly.

In addition, because it is stored in adipose tissue and then gradually released, TD fentanyl may not be reliable in cachectic patients, who may find themselves on large doses of TD fentanyl without actually receiving much of the medication. When transitioning a cachectic patient off of TD fentanyl to another opioid, the equianalgesic amount from Table 2.1 may need to be reduced by 80% or more because the patient may not have been receiving much of the medication, and the patient must be observed closely for under- or overdosing in the transition.

Last, fentanyl is sometimes given transmucosally for breakthrough cancer pain unrelieved by other opioids. When dosing transmucosal fentanyl preparations as a prn medication, always start at the lowest available dosage regardless of the baseline regimen.[7] The rules for prescribing transmucosal fentanyl medication should not be considered the same as for other opioids in terms of the ratio between the total daily dosage and the breakthrough dose. Immediate-release PO and buccal fentanyl preparations are expensive and have unique properties with which prescribers should become familiar before prescribing. Usually other short-acting opioids are preferable for breakthrough prescribing when using TD fentanyl as a baseline medication.

Methadone

Methadone is a potent opioid with several favorable characteristics, including oral bioavailability of 80%, no active metabolites requiring dose adjustments in renal impairment, low cost, a steady analgesic effect, and (possibly) more efficacy than other opioids when used for neuropathic pain.[8] However, methadone has a long, variable half-life ranging from 6 to 190 hours, depending on the dosage. The rapid titration guidelines used for other opioids do not apply to methadone; in general, do not increase dosage more frequently than every 4 days in lower doses and 1 to 2 weeks in higher doses. Small changes in total daily dosage may slowly and progressively have a larger effect on blood level when patients are on dosages greater than 30 mg per day. Dose-conversion ratios are complex and vary based on current opioid dosage and individual factors (see Table 2.1). Such challenges of initial dosing and titration should not discourage providers from using methadone, provided they get assistance from specialists in pain management or palliative care if needed.

Because of the potential for drug accumulation from the long half-life in higher doses, always write "hold for sedation" when initially prescribing or changing dosages of methadone.

Converting from methadone back to morphine or other opioids is especially complex because methadone has a variable, often long half-life, and it affects more opioid receptors than other opioid analgesics; assistance from palliative care or pain management experts generally is advisable for this transition if patients have been on more than 30 mg of methadone for more than a few weeks.

Under most circumstances, unless the prescriber is very familiar with methadone pharmacokinetics, it is safer to use a different opioid with a much shorter half-life as a prn medication when using methadone as the baseline opioid. The usual calculation ratios and intervals used for determining breakthrough doses of other opioids do not apply to methadone (or fentanyl). Because of its long half-life, methadone is better used as a baseline, scheduled analgesic, with shorter-acting opioids, such as morphine or hydromorphone, used prn. In relatively stable situations, however, small doses of methadone can be given prn in addition to the scheduled regimen. In general, no matter how high the regular standing methadone dosage, the prn dosage should be no more than 2.5 mg to 5 mg two or three times daily. Because of the progressively long half-life, small incremental doses in patients receiving a large baseline dose may have a major effect on blood level if taken regularly. (Note. The longer half-life in larger doses does not mean that the analgesic effect also will be prolonged. The analgesic effect usually wears off at 8 to 12 hours, so dosing for pain should always be at least three times a day, even when high total doses are used.[9])

Although the ratio of PO methadone to IV methadone may vary from 1:1 to 2:1, when converting from PO to IV methadone, it is prudent to reduce the total daily dose of methadone by 50%. On the other hand, when converting from IV methadone to PO methadone, using the most conservative 1:1 conversion is recommended to avoid overmedicating the patient. In these transitions, the patient should be carefully observed for under- and overdosing.

Cautions About Methadone

- As with any opioid, methadone may cause sedation, confusion, and respiratory depression, especially with rapid titration. Because of its long half-life, such adverse effects may not be apparent until several days after treatment initiation. If a patient does become oversedated, it may take many days for the sedative effects to wear off, depending on the dose.
- Methadone in moderate to high dosages can prolong the QTc interval and increase the risk of the potentially lethal *torsades de pointes*

arrhythmia.[10] Depending on a patient's prognosis and goals of care, consider checking the QTc at baseline, and begin monitoring after each dosage change for patients taking more than 60 mg of methadone per day. If QTc becomes significantly prolonged (QTc 450-499 milliseconds = moderate risk; QTc > 500 milliseconds = high risk), consideration should be given to lowering the methadone dosage or rotating to an alternate opioid. Patients with predisposing factors for arrhythmia (electrolyte abnormalities, heart disease), those already on medications that affect QTc, or those on medications that decrease methadone clearance may require more vigilant monitoring. Formal consultation with palliative care, acute pain service, cardiology, and pharmacy should be considered.

- Medications that can decrease methadone levels include rifampin, phenytoin, corticosteroids, carbamazepine, phenobarbital, St. John's Wort, and a number of antiretroviral agents.
- Medications that can increase methadone levels include tricyclic antidepressants, azole antifungals (especially voriconazole), macrolides and fluoroquinolones, amiodarone, and selective serotonin reuptake inhibitors. Use caution when prescribing benzodiazepines if a patient is on methadone because of the additive risk of oversedation.

Sample Calculation 2. Conversion to Methadone

A 50-year-old woman with metastatic breast cancer has good pain control with two sustained-release 200 mg PO morphine tablets twice a day. However, she develops persistent myoclonus. Because she is able to swallow pills and would prefer to stay on a longer-acting medication, you decide to rotate from morphine to methadone. (The conversion table [Table 2.1] always requires that the equianalgesic amount of oral morphine be determined to calculate a daily dosage of methadone, even if the patient is initially on a different opioid.)

Step 1. Calculate the total daily oral morphine dosage.
- Two tablets of 200 mg each taken twice daily = 800 mg total PO morphine per day

Step 2. Convert to methadone.

- For a dosage of 800 mg per day, the conversion ratio of morphine to methadone is 15:1 (see Table 2.1).
- 800 mg per day oral morphine × 1 mg methadone/15 mg PO morphine = 53 mg methadone per day

Step 3. Reduce the dosage because of incomplete cross-tolerance.

- Because her pain in currently well controlled, you reduce the equi-analgesic dose by one-third to one-half when switching to methadone because of incomplete cross-tolerance.
- 53 mg × ⅔ = about 35 mg methadone; alternatively, 53 mg × ½ = about 26 mg methadone
- Total daily dosage should be between 26 mg and 35 mg methadone per day.
- The baseline methadone dosage should be increased no more frequently than every 4 to 7 days because of the danger of gradual accumulation.

Step 4. Determine dosing schedule.

- Methadone is initially given in divided doses three times per day because of the limited duration of the analgesic effect, even when its half-life may be considerably longer.
- A dosage of 30 mg (between 26 mg and 35 mg) of methadone per day can be given as 10 mg three times per day.
- When ordering methadone, because of its long and variable half-life, always write "*hold for sedation.*"

Step 5. Choose a prn medication.

- Because of its potentially long half-life, prn doses of methadone can be difficult to manage correctly. Therefore, an opioid with a short half-life is generally preferable for prn dosing.

Step 6. Determine the prn dose (morphine).

- The prn dose should typically be 10% of the total daily opioid dosage.
- Because the patient was already on 800 mg per day of PO morphine, the prn dose based on the prior total daily dosage of morphine

would be 800 mg PO morphine × 10% = 80 mg PO morphine every 1 to 2 hours prn.

- Because she has an oral route, the morphine can be administered as 4 mL of 20 mg/mL morphine concentrate or equivalent every 1 to 2 hours prn.

2C | Treatment of Acute Pain Crisis

A pain crisis is an event in which a patient reports intense, uncontrolled pain that is causing severe personal or family distress.[11] Such a crisis may represent an acute change in the patient's condition, or it may result from gradually increasing pain that crosses a threshold and becomes intolerable. Usually, patients rate this pain as 7/10 to 10/10, and it dominates all other experiences. Acute pain crisis should be treated as a palliative care emergency.

The first step in managing such a crisis is to make a careful patient assessment. The extent of the work-up will be determined to a large extent by the patient's underlying disease, prognosis, prior functional status, preferences, and past pain experiences and behavior. In all circumstances, the work-up begins with a careful history and physical examination. If the pain heralds an abrupt change in clinical status, evaluation may include diagnostic procedures, especially if the results will lead to potentially effective treatments that would improve the patient's quality of life and be acceptable to him or her. If there is uncertainty about the efficacy of an invasive measure or why the current pain regimen has become ineffective, consultation from palliative care or acute pain service can be helpful.

While the patient is being evaluated for specific interventions that may help, an opioid bolus of 10% of the total daily dose can be given. Efficacy should be assessed in 10 to 15 minutes: If pain is still present, a higher dose (increased 25% to 50% for moderate to severe pain) can be administered. Subsequent doses can be given every 15 minutes until adequate analgesia is obtained. Once the effective dose is found, it can be scheduled to be given every 4 hours (assuming normal renal and hepatic function).[3]

If the prior opioid dosage has been rapidly and substantially increased over a short period and tolerance is suspected, the equianalgesic amount of any new opioid may need to be reduced substantially.

In all of these situations in which there is an acute pain crisis, the treating team should carefully and frequently observe the patient, making adjustments continually until the pain reaches at least a moderate level.

2D | General Opioid Side Effects and Caveats[12]

Respiratory Depression

Except for patients who are chronic carbon dioxide (CO_2) retainers, clinically significant respiratory depression is rare when opioid dosages are carefully titrated. Respiratory diseases such as congestive heart failure, chronic obstructive pulmonary disease, and lung cancer should not be barriers to opioid use; opioids provide these patients with the additional benefit of relieving dyspnea (see chapter 3). Furthermore, respiratory depression almost always is preceded by sedation; cutting back on the dosage if sedation develops usually avoids respiratory depression. For patients at risk for CO_2 retention, starting doses should be halved and baseline treatment should always start with short-acting medications.

Constipation

Opioids decrease bowel motility, so constipation develops in almost all patients on chronic opioids. When starting an opioid, prescribe a bowel regimen such as senna or bisacodyl, or an osmotic agent such as polyethylene glycol, sorbitol, or lactulose (see chapter 4 for a wider range of options and dosages). Although docusate sodium can be used in addition to a laxative, in general it is not effective as a single agent for opioid-induced constipation. Fiber supplements should be avoided in patients prone to dehydration or those with impaired mobility because of the risk of pseudo-obstruction.

Nausea

Nausea may occur with the initiation of opioids but usually resolves after several days as the patient develops tolerance to this side effect. If it remains persistent after the initiation of a new opioid medication, make sure the patient is not constipated, look for other drug interactions, and then consider dosage reduction or opioid rotation (see chapter 4).

Sedation

Mild sedation is relatively common when first starting an opioid and also when making significant dosage adjustments upward. Tolerance to the sedating effects of opioids usually develops rapidly (if given on a scheduled basis), whereas the analgesic effect persists. It is important to educate patients about the temporary nature of mild sedation when they are starting opioids because this may improve compliance. Tolerance to sedating effects is less likely to occur with infrequent or prn-only use. If sedation continues, a psychostimulant can be added to try to improve alertness, depending on the clinical situation.

Myoclonus

Some patients on opioids develop uncontrolled, intermittent twitching. It usually can be managed by checking for electrolyte abnormalities (if appropriate), reducing the dosage, rotating opioids, or adding benzodiazepines.

Delirium

Delirium can be caused or aggravated by opioids, especially in older adults or patients with underlying metabolic problems. This can usually be managed by dosage reduction, opioid rotation, or separate treatment of the associated delirium as described in chapter 5. On the other hand, untreated pain can precipitate or exacerbate delirium. Therefore, a careful pain assessment and sometimes a therapeutic trial of opioids may be warranted.

History of Intolerable Side Effects

If patients have had severe adverse effects from opioids in the past (eg, respiratory depression, seizures, delirium), the particular opioids associated with the adverse effects should be avoided, and other opioids should be used with caution (ie, start with a very low dosage) if clearly indicated. However, a past history of milder side effects, such as sedation or nausea, is common; such symptoms often are time limited and can be managed by opioid dosage reduction, rotation, or other symptom-targeted therapies (eg, adding an antiemetic before each opioid dose for the first 2 days to prevent nausea).

Urinary Retention

Low urine output or symptoms of suprapubic pain after initiating opioid therapy can indicate opioid-induced urinary retention. Review the patient's medication list and past medical history for other possible culprits, such as a history of prostatic enlargement or use of anticholinergic medications. Urinary retention in a patient with back pain, advanced cancer, an abnormal neurologic exam, or known vertebral metastases may indicate spinal cord compression (although bowel or bladder dysfunction is a late finding).

2E | Addiction and Abuse

There has been an epidemic of prescription drug abuse in the United States that has worsened in the last 10 years.[1] All clinicians who potentially prescribe opioids for acute or chronic pain should be aware of the potential risk factors for abuse and vigilant in identifying and responding to warning signs of opioid misuse (asking for early refills, lost prescriptions, repeated requests for dose escalation, obtaining prescriptions from multiple sources). Risk factors include

- a personal or family history of alcohol or drug abuse
- a personal or family history of a major psychiatric disorder
- poor socioeconomic status.

The presence of risk factors should not preclude the use of opioid analgesia in a palliative care setting, especially in the presence of severe progressive illness, but such prescribing requires written prescribing contracts.[13] Palliative care or addiction medicine consultation should be considered in this situation. Some have argued that prescribing contracts should be used for all patients on chronic opioids because of the difficulty of reliably identifying all who are at risk of misuse and to avoid the stigma of using contracts with some and not others. Key elements of prescribing contracts include

- a single designated prescriber and pharmacy for any and all controlled substances
- strictly limited supplies of controlled substances
- no early refills or dose changes by anyone other than the designated prescriber
- regular face-to-face meetings for refills
- random drug testing for the presence of the prescribed medication and absence of other substances of abuse
- clear education about not sharing medications and safe storage
- clearly enforced consequences for violating elements of the contract.

Although all opioids have the potential to be abused, both short- and long-acting oxycodone seem particularly susceptible and should be avoided in patients who are at risk for abuse.

In thinking about abuse, remember the following distinctions[14]:

- *Addiction* is characterized by impaired control over drug use, craving, compulsive use, use in unprescribed ways, and continued use despite harm.
- *Physical dependence* is manifested by a physiologic withdrawal syndrome that can be produced by abrupt cessation, rapid dosage reduction, decreasing blood level, or administration of an antagonist (eg, naloxone).
- *Tolerance* is a state of adaptation in which exposure to a drug induces changes that result in a diminution of one or more of the drug's effects over time. A patient who has become tolerant may report inadequate pain relief with a previously effective opioid dosage and may require increasingly larger dosages over time to achieve the same effect. For many patients, one or two dosage adjustments over time are sufficient.

- *Pseudoaddiction* is an iatrogenic syndrome that mimics behaviors commonly associated with addiction. It occurs when inadequately treated pain leads to patient demands for opioids that care providers deem excessive, leading to distrust between the patient and medical staff. These potentially maladaptive behaviors disappear when pain is adequately controlled and medications are predictably available.

Both physical dependence and limited tolerance are seen in virtually all patients receiving chronic opioids and are not symptoms of abuse. The development of tolerance does not mean that adequate pain relief will not be achievable as symptoms escalate, as long as dosages are adjusted accordingly. Tolerance does not seem to cross classes of opioids, so changing to a different medication (opioid rotation) provides a sensible way to address increasing pain in a patient who has developed rapidly increasing tolerance. When switching from one opioid to another, the equianalgesic dosage needs to be adjusted downward (usually by 30% to 50%) because of incomplete cross-tolerance between opioids.

2F | Adjuvant Analgesia

Adjuvant analgesia includes pharmacologic and nonpharmacologic therapies that are often effective in treating pain. In clinical practice, adjuvants are frequently reserved for pain that does not respond well to opioids or to allow dosage reduction when side effects limit opioid use, but the World Health Organization recommends that adjuvant medications be considered at all levels of pain severity. Adjuvants should be considered before opioids for patients with chronic nonmalignant pain that is likely to be long lasting. Adjuvants should be targeted to the particular type of pain (neuropathic, somatic, visceral), and careful consideration should be given to balancing both desired effects and potential side effects. For moderate to severe pain, combination therapy with an opioid and an adjuvant can frequently achieve better pain relief with less toxicity than continued escalation of opioid monotherapy. Foremost among the adjuvant pharmacologic agents are specific antidepressants, anticonvulsants, anti-inflammatories, and topical agents.[15,16] The evidence base supporting specific selection of adjuvant agents is highly variable, but examples of commonly prescribed adjuvants combined with starting doses and some prescribing caveats are presented in **Table 2.2**. Prescribers who are unfamiliar with the combined use of these medications are encouraged to discuss their plans with specialists in palliative care or pain management.

2G | Procedural Methods of Pain Relief

Nerve blocks have a strong track record of effectiveness and safety in properly selected patients. They are particularly useful for deep visceral pain (eg, pancreatic cancer or liver metastases), but also local plexopathy-related pain. Formal and informal consultation with an interventional pain specialist may help determine whether there may be a role for interventional therapies such as spinal infusions; peripheral plexus catheters; and neuraxial blocks, both with local anesthetic infusions and neurolytics[17,18] (**Table 2.3**). If such techniques are employed, analgesic medications initially are continued unless they have caused adverse effects; often the analgesic dosage can be decreased if the invasive measure successfully reduces the pain. Keep in mind that a terminal illness does not preclude the use of invasive pain-relieving techniques if those interventions help improve functional status, physical symptoms, or other patient goals.

2H | Nonpharmacologic Methods

Many patients have reported improved relief from methods such as those in **Table 2.4**,[19] but there is little systematic research to guide their use. These methods often can be added to the pharmacologic methods discussed above.

Table 2.2 Selected Adjuvant Analgesic Drugs by Pain Type

DRUG CLASS	EXAMPLES: STARTING DOSE/ MAXIMUM†	NOTES
Somatic pain—aching, throbbing, stabbing; examples include bone metastases, wounds, soft tissue tumors, arthritis		
NSAIDs	Naproxen 500 mg PO, then 500 mg every 8 hours; max. 1,500 mg daily Ibuprofen 400 mg-800 mg every 6-8 hours; max. 3,200 mg daily	Can be limited by GI, renal, and cardiac effects; may exacerbate hemorrhagic conditions; avoid in renal or liver impairment; avoid use in older adults; periodically monitor blood pressure, blood urea nitrogen, creatinine, liver function tests, complete blood cell count, and fecal occult blood
Acetaminophen	Acetaminophen 325 mg-650 mg every 4-6 hours; maximum 4,000 mg daily	Excessive dosing leads to liver toxicity; monitor platelet and liver function with chronic disease; some regulators recommend a maximum dose of 3,000 mg per day because of the risk of unintentional overdose.[20]
Bisphosphonates[21]	Pamidronate 60 mg-90 mg infused over 90-120 minutes Zolendronate 4 mg over 15 minutes	Consensus guidelines recommend regular use to prevent fractures with osteolytic bone lesions from breast cancer, multiple myeloma and other solid tumors,[22-24] and for patients on long-term steroids.[25] Side effects include nausea, fever, renal dysfunction, hypocalcemia, and osteonecrosis of jaw. Effective for relief from bone metastases; higher dosage associated with increased creatinine
Corticosteroids[26]	Dexamethasone 1 mg-4 mg PO/SC/IV two to three times daily; maximum 16 mg per day; taper rapidly to the lowest dose that achieves the desired effect; avoid nighttime dosing if possible Prednisone 20 mg-30 mg PO two or three times per day (rapidly taper as tolerated)	Consider time-limited trial with clear goals and endpoints; short-term adverse effects include impaired glucose control, thrush, dyspepsia, insomnia, delirium, anxiety, hypertension, and immunosuppression; long-term side effects include Cushingoid habitus, proximal myopathy, osteoporosis, and aseptic necrosis.

Table 2.2 Selected Adjuvant Analgesic Drugs by Pain Type *continued*

DRUG CLASS	EXAMPLES: STARTING DOSE/ MAXIMUM[†]	NOTES
Neuropathic pain—burning, tingling, shooting, painful numbness; examples include postherpetic neuralgia, diabetic neuropathy, and compression radiculopathies[27-29]		
Tricyclic antidepressants	Nortriptyline or desipramine, start at 10-25 mg at hs; increase every 3-7 days as tolerated; nortriptyline maximum 150 mg/day; desipramine maximum 300 mg/day	Sedation, anticholinergic effects, cardiac arrhythmias; give initial dose at hs because of sedating effect; concurrent treatment of depression; avoid if patient already is too sleepy/lethargic
Selective serotonin and norepinephrine reuptake inhibitors	Venlafaxine 37.5 mg once daily; increase by 37.5 mg-75 mg weekly as tolerated; 225 mg per day maximum. Duloxetine, start at 30 mg daily; titrate to 60 mg after a week, if tolerated	Nausea; decrease dosage in patients with renal impairment (avoid duloxetine if CrCl <30 mL/min); use caution in patients with hepatic impairment
Anticonvulsants	Gabapentin 100 mg-300 mg PO at bedtime; increase as tolerated; max. dose 3,600 mg per day Pregabalin 25 mg-50 mg PO three times daily; max. 600 mg daily in divided doses	Sedation and dizziness; no major drug-drug interactions; decrease dosage in patients with renal impairment
Topical analgesics[30]	TD lidocaine patch 5%, 1-3 patches up to 12 hours per day	Caution in patients with advanced liver failure due to decreased clearance of lidocaine; anecdotal effectiveness in patients with somatic pain; few side effects other than rash or local erythema
	Capsaicin cream[31]	Peripheral neuropathic pain; some find burning sensation difficult to tolerate

continued

Table 2.2 Selected Adjuvant Analgesic Drugs by Pain Type *continued*

DRUG CLASS	EXAMPLES: STARTING DOSE/ MAXIMUM[†]	NOTES
Visceral pain—not well localized, cramping, colicky, pressure, spastic; examples include bowel obstruction, bulky liver metastases		
Anticholinergics[32]	Scopolamine 1 or 3 patches every 3 days	Can cause delirium, lethargy, constipation, urinary retention
	Hyoscyamine 0.125 mg-0.25 mg PO/SC/IV every 4 hours, max. 12 tabs per day	Same as above, but often better tolerated
	Glycopyrrolate 0.2 mg-0.4 mg IV or SC every 4 hours prn	Same as above, but often better tolerated

CrCl, creatine clearance; GI, gastrointestinal; hs, bedtime; IV, intravenous; PO, oral; SC, subcutaneous.

[†]*Dosages based on Weinstein SM, Portenoy RK, Harrington SE. C. Porter Storey, ed. UNIPAC 3: Assessing and Treating Pain. 4th ed. Glenview, IL: American Academy of Hospice and Palliative Medicine; 2012.*

Table 2.3 Select Procedural Methods of Pain Relief

METHOD	TYPE	INDICATION
Nerve blocks[17,18]	Peripheral nerve or plexus block	Used for somatic pain in discrete dermatomes (eg, mandibular nerve block for facial pain, intercostal block for chest wall pain, paravertebral block for radicular pain, and brachial plexus block for brachial plexus involvement)
	Celiac plexus	Used for pain originating from upper abdominal viscera: pancreas, gallbladder, liver, mesentery, GI tract from stomach to transverse colon, and adrenal glands
	Hypogastric plexus	Used for pain originating from pelvic viscera: descending and sigmoid colon, rectum, bladder, testes, uterus, and ovaries
	Ganglion impar	For pain originating from anorectal area or lower part of vagina
Spinal infusions[17,18]	Epidural opioid ± bupivacaine ± clonidine	Used for chest wall pain over several dermatomes, abdominal pain, lumbosacral, perineal pain, and lower extremity pain; ambulation can potentially be compromised for patients with lumbosacral and lower extremity involvement
	Intrathecal opioid ± bupivacaine ± clonidine	Same indications as for epidural pain, but potentially can be associated with more numbness and weakness
Surgery[33]	Neurosurgical ablative procedures (rarely indicated given availability and effectiveness of other options)	Cordotomy, trigeminal tractotomy
	Orthopedic procedures	Decompressive surgery for spinal cord metastases, hip fracture repair, and fracture fixation
	Vascular procedures	Stenting for peripheral arterial disease, amputation
External beam radiation therapy[34-36]	Shorter courses (1-5) with higher fractions should always be considered for patients with advanced disease	Used for painful bony, visceral, or cutaneous disease; spinal cord compression; brain metastases
		Effects generally are noticed within 2 weeks but may take up to 6 weeks for full effect
Radiopharmaceuticals[37]	Strontium-89, samarium-153, phosphorus-32	Used for multiple, painful osteoblastic lesions

Table 2.4 Nonpharmacologic Approaches to Pain Control

Use of specialized mattress and every-2-hour turning for pressure ulcers
Massage therapy
Biofeedback
Music
Distraction
Humor
Therapeutic touch
Chiropractic manipulation
Pet therapy
Transepidermal nerve stimulator unit
Acupuncture
Local heat or cold
Education about illness
Hypnosis
Guided imagery
Cognitive and behavioral therapies

Further Discussion

1. If using immediate-release morphine as a baseline medication to manage chronic pain, what would be the proper dosing interval?

2. Based on the time to peak effect, what is the best time interval to prescribe prn doses of immediate-release morphine given orally? How about parenterally?

3. What is the best method for estimating the size of a prn dosage of opioid based on the total daily opioid dose?

4. When changing from one opioid to another, what is incomplete cross-tolerance and how much should a calculated equianalgesic dose be adjusted accordingly?

5. How significant is the risk of respiratory depression when prescribing opioids? What is the relationship between sedation and respiratory depression?

6. How significant is the risk of constipation when prescribing opioids? How do you anticipate and treat this problem?

7. Define the following terms and estimate the prevalence of each condition in a palliative care setting.
   - Physical dependence
   - Tolerance
   - Addiction
   - Pseudoaddiction

Case Study

A man with metastatic prostate cancer rates his pain as 8/10 and is currently taking two oxycodone/acetaminophen (5/325) tablets every 4 hours around the clock. He needs better pain relief.

- Why not just increase the dose of oxycodone/acetaminophen?
- Using the equianalgesic table (Table 2.1), calculate the daily dose of oxycodone, increase it by one-third, and calculate a new dose and interval of short-acting oxycodone to use as his maintenance (around-the-clock) medication. Also calculate an appropriate prn dose and interval.

On day 3, his pain is improving and is now averaging a 4/10, which he finds acceptable. He has taken 25 mg of oxycodone every 4 hours and an average of four prn doses of 15 mg each day for the last several days. Unfortunately, he starts vomiting and has been made NPO. You decide to rotate opioids to IV morphine.

- Calculate an equianalgesic amount of IV morphine, and calculate an hourly rate and an appropriate prn dose. (Note. Don't forget to account for incomplete cross-tolerance.)

continued

His pain is eventually controlled, and the patient is discharged on 90 mg PO morphine twice a day. He is enrolled in hospice and does well before he develops excruciating back pain, which he describes as 10/10, associated with nausea and vomiting. You are not sure if the nausea and vomiting are from the morphine (his creatinine has now risen to 2.5 mg/dL) or from a medical complication of his illness, so you decide to rotate opioids to hydromorphone.

- Calculate an hourly rate of a hydromorphone drip and an appropriate prn dose and interval. (Note. Because his pain is poorly controlled, be sure to consider how you would increase the dose and how you would adjust for incomplete cross-tolerance.)

- Are there any diagnostic procedures that should be considered? Does the fact that he is enrolled in hospice limit diagnostic or therapeutic options for this patient?

After several opioid dose adjustments, treatment with steroids, and acute radiation to his spine, his pain is reported to be "mild." His parenteral dose of hydromorphone is 1.5 mg/hour, and he has not required any prn doses in the past 24 hours. You try a fentanyl patch as his baseline and use PO hydromorphone as his prn medication.

- What size patch would you use, and what is a proper prn dose of oral hydromorphone? (Please note the special considerations for incomplete cross-tolerance with fentanyl noted in the comments section of the equianalgesic card.)

He does well for several weeks on two 100-mcg patches/hour every 3 days, but recently his pain has increased with a strong neuropathic component (ie, lancinating, burning, jabbing quality). He is now taking four 8-mg hydromorphone tablets per day, and his pain is averaging 7/10. You have tried adding gabapentin and then pregabalin as adjuvant medications, but neither medication has helped. You consider methadone.

- Why might this be a good choice?

Calculate an initial starting dose of methadone based on his total daily dose of opioids. (Note. You will have to calculate a total daily dose equivalent of PO morphine to get to the methadone dose.)

- Because of methadone's long and variable half-life, it is not easy to use as a prn medication. Therefore, you decide to continue to use hydromorphone as his prn medication. What should be the dose and interval?

- Name three characteristics of methadone that make it a particularly attractive medication in the palliative care setting.

- Name three things about methadone that make it challenging to use in this setting.

- How frequently should his methadone dose be adjusted?

References

1. Dowell D, Kunins HV, Farley TA. Opioid analgesics—risky drugs, not risky patients. *JAMA*. 2013;309(21):2219-2220.

2. Dean M. Opioids in renal failure and dialysis patients. *J Pain Symptom Manage*. 2004;28(5):497-504.

3. Goldstein NE, Morrison RS. *Evidence-Based Practice of Palliative Medicine*. Philadelphia, PA: Saunders; 2013.

4. American Geriatric Society. Pharmacological management of persistent pain in older persons. *J Am Geriatr Soc*. 2009;57(8):1331-1346.

5. Fine PG, Portenoy RK. Establishing "best practices" for opioid rotation: conclusions of an expert panel. *J Pain Symptom Manage*. 2009;38(3):418-425.

6. Knotkova H, Fine PG, Portenoy RK. Opioid rotation: the science and the limitations of the equianalgesic dose table. *J Pain Symptom Manage*. 2009;38(3):426-439.

7. Portenoy RK, Taylor D, Messina J, Tremmel L. A randomized, placebo-controlled study of fentanyl buccal tablet for breakthrough pain in opioid-treated patients with cancer. *Clin J Pain*. 2006;22(9):805-811.

8. Morley JS, Bridson J, Nash TP, Miles JB, White S, Makin MK. Low-dose methadone has an analgesic effect in neuropathic pain: a double-blind randomized controlled crossover trial. *Palliat Med.* 2003;17(7):576-587.

9. Davis MP, Walsh D. Methadone for relief of cancer pain: a review of pharmacokinetics, pharmacodynamics, drug interactions and protocols of administration. *Support Care Cancer.* 2001;9(2):73-83.

10. Krantz MJ, Martin J, Stimmel B, Mehta D, Haigney MC. QTc interval screening in methadone treatment. *Ann Intern Med.* 2009;150(6):387-395.

11. Moryl N, Coyle N, Foley KM. Managing an acute pain crisis in a patient with advanced cancer: "this is as much of a crisis as a code." *JAMA.* 2008;299(12):1457-1467.

12. Labianca R, Sarzi-Puttini P, Zuccaro SM, Cherubino P, Vellucci R, Fornasari D. Adverse effects associated with non-opioid and opioid treatment in patients with chronic pain. *Clin Drug Investig.* 2012;32 Suppl 1:53-63.

13. Passik SD, Portenoy RK, Ricketts PL. Substance abuse issues in cancer patients. Part 2: Evaluation and treatment. *Oncology (Williston).* 1998;12(5):729-734; discussion 736, 741-722.

14. Passik SD, Portenoy RK, Ricketts PL. Substance abuse issues in cancer patients. Part 1: Prevalence and diagnosis. *Oncology (Williston).* 1998;12(4):517-521, 524.

15. Dworkin RH, O'Connor AB, Audette J, et al. Recommendations for the pharmacological management of neuropathic pain: an overview and literature update. *Mayo Clin Proc.* 2010;85(3 Suppl):S3-14.

16. Moulin DE, Clark AJ, Gilron I, et al. Pharmacological management of chronic neuropathic pain—consensus statement and guidelines from the Canadian Pain Society. *Pain Res Manag.* 2007;12(1):13-21.

17. Christo PJ, Mazloomdoost D. Interventional pain treatments for cancer pain. *Ann N Y Acad Sci.* 2008;1138:299-328.

18. Kaplan R, Portenoy RK. Cancer pain management: interventional therapies. *Up To Date.* 2011;Version 19.3.

19. Blaes AH, Kreitzer MJ, Torkelson C, Haddad T. Nonpharmacologic complementary therapies in symptom management for breast cancer survivors. *Semin Oncol.* 2011;38(3):394-402.

20. US Food and Drug Administration. Prescription acetamenophen products to be limited to 325 mg per dosage unit: boxed warning will highlight potential for severe liver failure. 2013. www.fda.gov/Drugs/DrugSafety/ucm239821.htm. Accessed July 20, 2013.

21. Weinstein E, Arnold R. Bisphosphonates for bone pain. *Fast Facts and Concepts #113*. End of Life/ Palliative Education Resource Center; 2009. Available at www.mcw.edu/FileLibrary/User/jrehm/fastfactpdfs/Concept113.pdf. Accessed December 15, 2013.

22. Aapro M, Abrahamsson PA, Body JJ, et al. Guidance on the use of bisphosphonates in solid tumours: recommendations of an international expert panel. *Ann Oncol*. 2008;19(3):420-432.

23. Cuzick J, DeCensi A, Arun B, et al. Preventive therapy for breast cancer: a consensus statement. *Lancet Oncol*. 2011;12(5):496-503.

24. Hillner BE, Ingle JN, Berenson JR, et al. American Society of Clinical Oncology guideline on the role of bisphosphonates in breast cancer. American Society of Clinical Oncology Bisphosphonates Expert Panel. *J Clin Oncol*. 2000;18(6):1378-1391.

25. Stoch SA, Saag KG, Greenwald M, et al. Once-weekly oral alendronate 70 mg in patients with glucocorticoid-induced bone loss: a 12-month randomized, placebo-controlled clinical trial. *J Rheumatol*. 2009;36(8):1705-1714.

26. Weinstein E AR. Steriods in the treatment of bone pain. *Fast Facts and Concepts #129*. End of Life/ Palliative Education Resource Center; 2009. www.mcw.edu/FileLibrary/User/jrehm/fastfactpdfs/Concept129.pdf. Accessed October 20, 2013.

27. McGeeney BE. Pharmacological management of neuropathic pain in older adults: an update on peripherally and centrally acting agents. *J Pain Symptom Manage*. 2009;38(2 Suppl):S15-27.

28. Saarto T, Wiffen PJ. Antidepressants for neuropathic pain: a Cochrane review. *J Neurol Neurosurg Psychiatry*. 2010;81(12):1372-1373.

29. Rutkove SB. A 52-year-old woman with disabling peripheral neuropathy: review of diabetic polyneuropathy. *JAMA*. 2009;302(13):1451-1458.

30. Rosielle D. The lidocaine patch. *Fast Facts and Concepts #148*. End of Life/ Palliative Education Resource Center; 2009. Available at www.mcw.edu/FileLibrary/User/jrehm/fastfactpdfs/Concept148.pdf.

31. Knotkova H, Pappagallo M, Szallasi A. Capsaicin (TRPV1 Agonist) therapy for pain relief: farewell or revival? *Clin J Pain*. 2008;24(2):142-154.

32. Mercadante S, Casuccio A, Mangione S. Medical treatment for inoperable malignant bowel obstruction: a qualitative systematic review. *J Pain Symptom Manage*. 2007;33(2):217-223.

33. Patchell RA, Tibbs PA, Regine WF, et al. Direct decompressive surgical resection in the treatment of spinal cord compression caused by metastatic cancer: a randomized trial. *Lancet*. 2005;366:643-648.

34. Chow E, Harris K, Fan G, Tsao M, Sze WM. Palliative radiotherapy trials for bone metastases: a systematic review. *J Clin Oncol*. 2007;25(11):1423-1436.

35. Fairchild A, Barnes E, Ghosh S, et al. International patterns of practice in palliative radiotherapy for painful bone metastases: evidence-based practice? *Int J Radiat Oncol Biol Phys*. 2009;75(5):1501-1510.

36. Janjan N, Lutz ST, Bedwinek JM, et al. Therapeutic guidelines for the treatment of bone metastasis: a report from the American College of Radiology Appropriateness Criteria Expert Panel on Radiation Oncology. *J Palliat Med*. May 2009;12(5):417-426.

37. Reisfield G, Wilson G. Radiopharmaceuticals for painful osseous metastases. *Fast Facts and Concepts #116*. End of Life/ Palliative Education Resource Center; 2004. Available at www.eperc.mcw.edu/EPERC/ FastFactsIndex/ff_116.htm.

THREE

Dyspnea

Dyspnea is defined by the American Thoracic Society as "a subjective experience of breathing discomfort."[1] Dyspnea is a distressing symptom that requires careful evaluation and urgent intervention when symptoms are severe. Unfortunately, dyspnea is a common symptom at the end of life, experienced by a majority of terminally ill cancer patients at some point during their illness.[2] Besides pulmonary and nonpulmonary malignancy, dyspnea can be caused by congestive heart failure (CHF), respiratory muscle weakness, chronic obstructive pulmonary disease (COPD), and several other etiologies (**Table 3.1**). Because of its subjective nature, dyspnea must be assessed by patient report. Respiratory rate or oxygen saturation levels may not accurately reflect symptom severity. Like pain, dyspnea should be assessed using validated measurement scales and followed sequentially as it is treated.

3A | Etiology

The initial step in treating dyspnea is to identify and, if possible, treat the underlying problem, be it COPD, cancer, CHF, pulmonary fibrosis, superior vena cava (SVC) syndrome, or pneumonitis (Table 3.1). Once these causes have been addressed with any available disease-directed therapies, the focus becomes palliative treatment of dyspnea as a symptom. Even with appropriate therapies for underlying disease, dyspnea sometimes remains a prominent and burdensome symptom. In general, this symptom can be significantly improved with proper treatment.

3B | General Treatment Measures

After the underlying etiology is addressed, several general measures can help alleviate dyspnea.
- Reduce the need for exertion.
- Reposition the patient to a more upright position.

- Keep the compromised lung down in unilateral disease.
- Improve air circulation by opening windows and doors or using a fan.
- Adjust humidity with a humidifier or air conditioner.
- Avoid strong odors, fumes, and smoke.
- Identify and avoid any triggers that precipitate or exacerbate dyspnea.
- Help the patient and family formulate a response plan if symptoms worsen.

Table 3.1 Common Etiologies of Dyspnea with Advanced Illness and Specific Disease-Directed Treatments

ETIOLOGY	TREATMENT
COPD	Bronchodilators (β2-agonists and anticholinergics), inhaled corticosteroids, and oxygen as appropriate
	Consider systemic corticosteroids for refractory symptoms.
CHF	Diuretics, ACE inhibitors, inotropes, vasodilators, angiotensin receptor blockers, beta-blockers
	Evaluate for potential left ventricular assist device (LVAD) or for cardiac transplant.
	Consider reducing or stopping artificial feedings or IV fluids.
Pneumonia	Consider whether antibiotics will meet the patient's goals; if patient circumstances are uncertain, consider a time-limited trial of antibiotics (patient and family participation in this decision is essential).
	If aspiration is suspected, diet can be modified (some patients choose an unrestricted diet to enjoy their favorite foods).
	Upright position during meals and careful hand feeding can limit risk.
	PEG tubes generally do not reduce the risk of aspiration.
Secretions	Thick secretions can be loosened with nebulized saline.
	Copious secretions can be reduced with anticholinergic medications (see **Table 3.3**).
Pain	Use appropriate pain management (as discussed in chapter 2).
Anxiety	Breathlessness can precipitate anxiety, and anxiety can worsen breathlessness; opioids generally are the first-line treatment in relieving breathlessness and are sometimes supplemented with anxiolytic therapy.

Table 3.1 Common Etiologies of Dyspnea with Advanced Illness and Specific Disease-Directed Treatments *continued*

ETIOLOGY	TREATMENT
Pleural effusion	Thoracentesis can be effective, though effusions often re-accumulate.
	Insertion of a tunneled drainage catheter is an option in the case of a recurring effusion and generally does not require hospitalization.
Anemia	Depending on the etiology and prognosis, a blood transfusion may temporarily reduce dyspnea; transfusions may be limited by CHF. When hemorrhage or marrow failure is part of the dying process, the associated dyspnea (from anemia) is best palliated with opioids and emotional and spiritual support.
Respiratory muscle weakness	Can be caused by deconditioning, cachexia, or motor neuron diseases (such as ALS); treat symptomatically
	Consider CPAP or tracheostomy and mechanical ventilation, depending on the goals of care.
Ascites	Consider therapeutic paracentesis.
	Drainage catheter placement sometimes is feasible when ascites re-accumulates rapidly, but may carry an increased risk of infection.
Pulmonary embolism	Weigh risks and benefits of anticoagulation (and its monitoring) according to patient goals and stage of disease.
SVC syndrome	Use oxygen, diuretics, elevation of head of the bed, and steroids. Consider palliative radiation therapy or pericardial window, depending on the clinical situation.
Malignant central airway obstruction	Depending on the clinical situation and patient goals, consider reducing tumor size via debulking surgery or radiation therapy, laser resection or tracheobronchial stenting, or perhaps even tracheostomy.
Pneumothorax	Consider a chest tube if it is consistent with the goals of care.
Pulmonary fibrosis	Use symptomatic treatment.

ACE, angiotensin-converting enzyme; ALS, amyotrophic lateral sclerosis; CHF, congestive heart failure; COPD, chronic obstructive pulmonary disease; CPAP, continuous positive airway pressure; IV, intravenous; PEG, percutaneous endoscopic gastrostomy; SVC, superior vena cava.

Opioid Therapy

Opioids are the preferred agents for symptomatically treating dyspnea because they effectively suppress awareness of the sensation of shortness of breath. They can be used alone or alongside treatment of reversible etiologies. Individually titrated, opioids have repeatedly been shown to be safe and effective in the treatment of dyspnea caused by cancer, COPD, pulmonary fibrosis, and CHF.[3] They generally are most beneficial for dyspnea at rest; when patients have dyspnea with exertion, a few minutes of rest usually resolves breathlessness faster than locating and administering a medication. Low dosages of oral or parenteral morphine usually provide relief for opioid-naïve patients; higher dosages may be needed for patients on chronic opioids. Acute, severe dyspnea should be treated with parenteral opioids in dosages titrated to reduce the patient's dyspnea to mild to moderate severity. For patients who cannot self-report, clinicians should monitor both the patient's facial expressions and respiratory rate in the assessment of respiratory distress, and adjust the opioid dosage accordingly. Continuous opioid infusion with additional patient-controlled analgesia (PCA) doses can be an effective method for treating severe dyspnea for patients capable of self-administration in the inpatient and outpatient setting. Nearly all routes of administration are effective, however evidence does not support the use of nebulized opioids.[4,5] Opioids are sometimes supplemented with anxiolytics for patients who remain anxious after the sensation of dyspnea has been properly treated with opioids. If opioid dosage is limited by drowsiness, reduce the benzodiazepine and, if needed, increase the opioid. There is emerging evidence (mainly in patients with COPD) that low dose (10 mg to 20 mg daily), sustained-release morphine may provide lasting relief of dyspnea.[6] It is not yet known how this approach compares to using short-acting agents around the clock. Type, route, and dosage of opioid should be decided on a case-by-case basis (**Table 3.2**).[7]

Some providers hesitate to use opioids for dyspnea because they fear respiratory depression. In the absence of pre-existing carbon dioxide (CO_2) retention, respiratory depression is uncommon and usually clinically insignificant in patients who are on carefully titrated or stable dosages of opioids. In patients with known CO_2 retention, starting doses should be halved and only short-acting opioids used until the patient's response is fully evaluated. Respiratory depression is almost always preceded by drowsiness; when ordering opioids for dyspnea, it is usually appropriate to specify "hold for sedation." Naloxone should be used only in emergent situations when life-threatening opioid toxicity is suspected (see chapter 2).

Table 3.2 Opioid Dosing for Management of Dyspnea

OPIOID TOLERANCE	DOSAGE
Opioid naïve	5 mg PO morphine equivalent as single dose; if tolerated, can administer every 4 hours around the clock, hold for sedation; an additional dose every hour in between scheduled doses can be made available prn for severe dyspnea.
Older adults, CO_2 retainers, or patients with renal impairment	Consider reducing starting dose by half. Avoid use of morphine in renal disease.
If current opioid dosage is inadequate	Titrate by increments of 25% to 50% to effect.
Dyspnea with exertion or movement	Give 30 minutes prior to activity.
If acutely dyspneic or actively dying	Use IV morphine bolus (2 mg-5 mg or 10% of daily dosage) every 5-10 minutes prn, titrate to effect (decline of self-reported dyspnea on 10-point scale); consider starting a continuous infusion based on the dosage needed to improve the patient's symptoms. For patients who cannot self-report, an improvement of non-verbal signs of distress or a decline in elevated respiratory rate toward the normal range may be used as surrogate markers of dyspnea.
If on stable opioid dosage	Consider a trial of a scheduled short-acting opioid or long-acting opioid as baseline, with immediate-release opioid prn in between.

IV, intravenous; CO_2, carbon dioxide; PO, oral; prn, as needed.

From Brown DJ. Palliation of breathlessness. Clin Med. 2006;6:133-136. ©2006 Royal College of Physicians. Adapted with permission.

Anxiolytic Therapy

Anxiety and dyspnea frequently exacerbate one another. Generally, treat an anxious, dyspneic patient with opioids first to reduce breathlessness, then follow with a benzodiazepine if needed.[8] Anxiety is often worse at night when patients have less social support. Oral lorazepam is a good choice to treat anxiety because of its relatively short half-life. It also is available as a liquid and can be administered sublingually for patients who have difficulty swallowing tablets. In patients with significant, persistent anxiety, scheduled dosing of a benzodiazepine is warranted, along with as-needed (prn) doses. Those with milder anxiety may find prn doses alone to be adequate. Parenteral benzodiazepines can be useful in the terminal phase, either given as intermittent boluses or via continuous infusion. Be sure to assess the anxious patient for depression, as these conditions often coexist. See chapter 5 for more detailed information about the treatment of both anxiety and depression.

Corticosteroids

Corticosteroids can reduce dyspnea in COPD, endotracheal malignancy, lymphangitic spread of cancer, pneumonitis, and SVC syndrome by reducing edema via their anti-inflammatory effects. Dexamethasone is often used and can be dosed 4 mg four times daily initially (with the evening dose administered in early evening to avoid insomnia), then reduced to a lower dose as tolerated for maintenance therapy. Any benefit should be noticed within a matter of days.[4] Watch for and address associated aggravation of anxiety or agitation.

Nonpharmacologic Measures

Nonpharmacologic measures are very helpful in addressing anxiety related to dyspnea. Sitting upright, using a bedside fan, listening to calming music, and practicing relaxation techniques can be effective, as can skillful counseling and the presence of calming caregivers. Pulmonary rehabilitation is worth considering for patients with COPD who are still ambulatory and can tolerate a more intensive exercise regimen. There is very limited evidence for complementary modalities such as acupuncture, but therapy should be tailored to the individual.[9]

Ventilatory Support

Noninvasive ventilatory support, ranging from supplemental oxygen to noninvasive positive pressure ventilation (NPPV), can be used to treat a dyspneic patient. Key points regarding noninvasive ventilatory support include the following:

- Dyspneic patients may like the sensation of air blowing on their face and obtain relief from low-flow oxygen or compressed air via nasal cannula. Watch for uncomfortable dryness of nasal passages and use moisturizing agents or humidification if needed.

- Although supplemental oxygen can reduce dyspnea in hypoxic COPD patients, its benefits are less established for cancer patients and may cause CO_2 retention in patients with amyotrophic lateral sclerosis (ALS).

- Unless the patient finds that breathing with a mask is more comfortable, face masks generally should be avoided because they can be frightening, cause feelings of isolation, and interfere with activities such as eating.

- Patients with COPD may find that NPPV increases their quality of life by reducing dyspnea and helping to preserve mental function as long as possible. Other patients find these devices too uncomfortable or anxiety provoking. Healthcare providers should weigh the pros and cons of such treatment on a case-by-case basis.

- For patients who can tolerate it, NPPV can be used to improve quality of life and possibly prolong survival in patients with dyspnea and chronic hypoventilation in neuromuscular disorders, particularly ALS patients with good bulbar function.[10]

The question of invasive ventilatory support comes up often for patients with advanced pulmonary disease. These questions should be resolved on a case-by-case basis, depending on the potential reversibility of patients' underlying illnesses as well as their personal goals and values. If invasive ventilatory support is contemplated, consider approaching its use as a time-limited trial.[11] The elements of a time-limited trial include

- specific time frame for reevaluating the intervention (days to weeks)
- agreed-upon markers for continuing or stopping therapy (such as continuing therapy if it results in improved quality of life or stopping it if quality declines)
- reassessment of the intervention according to the established time frame.

3C | Dyspnea in the Imminently Dying

When patients are actively dying, their weakness and mental status changes may make usual methods for assessing dyspnea less effective. If the patient loses the ability to report dyspnea, look for indicators such as nonverbal signs of distress (eg, grimacing, gasping) and ask the patient's caregivers for their assessment.[12] Providers may also follow the respiratory rate, but it is important not to confuse Cheyne-Stokes or Kussmaul respirations with a steady, rapid rate of breathing. For severe respiratory distress, the opioid dosage should be increased until the patient reports being more comfortable, or if unable to report, until the patient appears relatively comfortable and the respiratory rate approaches the normal range (20 or less). Once this is achieved, the opioid dosage should be continued at this level. Scheduled dosing should be used because actively dying patients typically cannot ask for prn doses due to sedation; prn doses should remain available for caregivers to administer if there are periodic, short-lived exacerbations. Dying patients with mild to moderate dyspnea can be treated with opioids via PO or sublingual (SL) routes. Those with more severe, uncontrolled symptoms of dyspnea should receive IV or SC opioids titrated rapidly to relief.

Because of concerns about these medical interventions potentially hastening death under these circumstances, it is critical to talk with staff and family about the purpose of the intervention (to relieve serious physical distress, not to hasten death) and the moral imperative for clinicians to be responsive to severe suffering in dying patients. Bedside clinicians responsible for carrying out these orders should be encouraged to voice their concerns, and any who still feel incapable of providing needed treatment should be assigned to other patients, if possible. By giving staff parameters to follow as they titrate opioid dosages (getting self-reported or caregiver-reported dyspnea severity down to 5 or below on a 10-point scale or getting the respiratory rate down to 20 instead of 40) helps create objective endpoints and alleviate some concerns about contributing to a patient's death. Severe shortness of breath is a palliative care emergency, and it is critical to have a team of providers committed to achieving adequate symptom relief.

3D | Continual Reassessment

Moderate to severe dyspnea constitutes a palliative care emergency that necessitates frequent reevaluation to determine if there is a need for different approaches to treatment. Reevaluate the need for

- adjustments in opioid dosage according to self-report of dyspnea on a 0 to 10 scale, or according to caregivers' assessment, nonverbal signals, and respiratory rate if the patient is unable to rate the sensation of dyspnea
- increased social, psychological, or spiritual support for patients and caregivers.[13]

Depending on the patient's stage of disease, associated symptoms, and goals, consider the addition of anxiolytics, corticosteroids, or antibiotics; or more invasive procedures, as discussed at beginning of this chapter.

3E | Respiratory Secretions

In addition to the loss of ability to take food and fluids, the process of dying impairs the cough/gag reflex and the ability to clear secretions and protect the airway from aspiration. The pooling of saliva in the posterior oropharynx and the retention of secretions in the tracheobronchial tree can lead to noisy respirations including gurgling, crackling, and rattling (sometimes referred to as the death rattle). To caregivers and family this can be quite disturbing and sound as though the patient is choking. Educating those involved in the patient's care is critical in the preparation for the last hours of life (see chapter 9); there is no evidence that these secretions are a source of distress for patients.

Nebulized saline may be helpful to loosen thick secretions but can also trigger coughing. Simple measures such as clearing food from the mouth or repositioning the patient for postural drainage can effectively relieve some symptoms. Nasopharyngeal or deep suctioning is rarely indicated, as this can cause considerable discomfort to the patient. In most cases, the secretions are located deeper in the respiratory tract and are not accessible to suctioning. Useful strategies for treating dyspnea also can be effective in relieving discomfort associated with the management of secretions.

Anticholinergic medications are the agents of choice for the treatment of copious secretions at the end of life, with no evidence for the superiority of one agent over another.[14,15] Atropine and scopolamine may cause varying degrees of confusion or delirium due to their ability to cross the blood-brain barrier (BBB). Glycopyrrolate and hyoscyamine do not cross the BBB and are less apt to cause these side effects. Dosing and route of administration for these medications is outlined in **Table 3.3**.

Table 3.3 Medications for Treatment of Oral Secretions at the End of Life

MEDICATION	STARTING DOSE/ ROUTE	TIME TO ONSET	NOTES
Atropine	1% ophthalmic drops, 1 or 2 drops SL every 1–2 hours prn	30 minutes	
Scopolamine	1 to 3 patches TD every 3 days, or 0.4 mg SC every 4–6 hours prn	12 hours (TD) 30 minutes (SC)	More than one patch may be used, but given time to onset, other medications should be considered if secretions persist.
Glycopyrrolate	0.2 mg-0.4 mg IV or SC every 4-8 hours prn	30 minutes (SC/IV)	More than one patch may be used, but given time to onset, other medications should be considered if secretions persist.
Hyoscyamine	0.125 mg orally disinte-grating tablets or 1 or 2 tablets PO or SL every 3–4 hours prn	20-30 minutes	Less likely than atro-pine or scopolamine to cause confusion.

IV, intravenous; PO, oral; prn, as needed; SC, subcutaneous; SL, sublingual; TD, transdermal.

Further Discussion

1. After all disease-specific measures to relieve dyspnea have been tried, name three nonpharmacological measures that might improve the sensation of dyspnea.

2. Most dyspneic patients are also anxious. What is the general approach to prescribing opioids and benzodiazepines in a seriously ill patient who is both dyspneic and anxious?

3. The management of dyspnea with opioids is similar to the management of pain with opioids (dosing intervals, calculating prn doses and intervals). Name two ways in which the management of dyspnea with opioids is different from their use in treating pain.

continued

An elderly man with advanced CHF on maximal medical therapy continues to be chronically short of breath despite careful efforts to maximize his treatment. He is not a transplant candidate and has refused treatment with IV inotropes. He understands that he might die soon and has completed do-not-resuscitate and do-not-intubate documents. His blood pressure is low (85/50), and he has significant renal insufficiency (creatinine 3.3 mg/dL).

- Which opioid should you avoid and why?
- You decide to start him on oral hydromorphone with around-the-clock and prn dosing. The patient is opioid naïve. What would be your starting dose of liquid hydromorphone? Calculate both maintenance and prn doses.

The patient is enrolled in hospice and hopes to be able to stay at home. You want to anticipate symptoms that might develop in the future and provide him with medications he may need at home.

- What would be your plan for managing potential dyspnea, anxiety, and respiratory secretions for a patient in their home? Consider exactly what you would write for each of the following symptoms:
  - Dyspnea
  - Anxiety
  - Respiratory secretions
- How might your management of dyspnea be different in a patient with known CO_2 retention?

Case Study 2

You are caring for an elderly woman with a history of metastatic lung cancer and delirium that has been difficult to manage. She is still periodically alert but has developed terminal secretions.

- What would be your medication of choice to treat her secretions and avoid exacerbating her delirium?

References

1. Parshall MB, Schwartzstein RM, Adams L, et al. An official American Thoracic Society statement: update on the mechanisms, assessment, and management of dyspnea. *Am J Respir Crit Care Med.* 2012;185(4):435-452.

2. Reuben DB, Mor V. Dyspnea in terminally ill cancer patients. *Chest.* 1986;89(2):234-236.

3. Kamal AH, Maguire JM, Wheeler JL, Currow DC, Abernethy AP. Dyspnea review for the palliative care professional: treatment goals and therapeutic options. *J Palliat Med.* 2012;15(1):106-114.

4. Del Fabbro E, Dalal S, Bruera E. Symptom control in palliative care–Part III: dyspnea and delirium. *J Palliat Med.* 2006;9(2):422-436.

5. LeGrand SB, Khawam EA, Walsh D, Rivera NI. Opioids, respiratory function, and dyspnea. *Am J Hosp Palliat Care.* 2003;20(1):57-61.

6. Currow DC, McDonald C, Oaten S, et al. Once-daily opioids for chronic dyspnea: a dose increment and pharmacovigilance study. *J Pain Symptom Manage.* 2011;42(3):388-399.

7. Brown DJ. Palliation of breathlessness. *Clin Med.* 2006;6(2):133-136.

8. Simon ST, Higginson IJ, Booth S, Harding R, Bausewein C. Benzodiazepines for the relief of breathlessness in advanced malignant and non-malignant diseases in adults. *Cochrane Database Syst Rev.* 2010(1):CD007354.

9. Bausewein C, Booth S, Gysels M, Higginson I. Non-pharmacological interventions for breathlessness in advanced stages of malignant and non-malignant diseases. *Cochrane Database Syst Rev.* 2008(2):CD005623.

10. Radunovic A, Annane D, Rafiq MK, Mustfa N. Mechanical ventilation for amyotrophic lateral sclerosis/motor neuron disease. *Cochrane Database Syst Rev.* 2013;3:CD004427.

11. Quill TE, Holloway R. Time-limited trials near the end of life. *JAMA.* 2011;306(13):1483-1484.

12. Hui D, Morgado M, Vidal M, et al. Dyspnea in hospitalized advanced cancer patients: subjective and physiologic correlates. *J Palliat Med.* 2013;16(3):274-280.

13. Malik FA, Gysels M, Higginson IJ. Living with breathlessness: a survey of caregivers of breathless patients with lung cancer or heart failure. *Palliat Med.* 2013;27(7):647-656.

14. Wee B, Hillier R. Interventions for noisy breathing in patients near to death. *Cochrane Database Syst Rev.* 2008(1):CD005177.

15. Wildiers H, Dhaenekint C, Demeulenaere P, et al. Atropine, hyoscine butylbromide, or scopolamine are equally effective for the treatment of death rattle in terminal care. *J Pain Symptom Manage.* 2009;38(1):124-133.

FOUR

Gastrointestinal Symptoms

4A | Common Oral Symptoms

Patients with life-limiting illnesses often have significant oral care needs that must be addressed to prevent and treat oral discomfort. These conditions also may be significant contributors to difficulty with swallowing (dysphagia). The palliative care team should be alert to the following syndromes (listed below with select etiologies) that often require specific interventions to improve symptoms:

Poor Oral Hygiene
- Patient weakness or depression
- Caregiver stress

Oral Pain
- Angular stomatitis (red fissures at the corners of the mouth, often from *Candida* or *Staphylococcal* infections)
- Dental caries or poorly fitting dentures
- Radiation- or chemotherapy-induced stomatitis or mucositis
- *Candidiasis* (white plaque, reddened tongue, or chronic multifocal candidiasis)
- Mucositis from other fungal, bacterial, or viral infections[1]
- Burning mouth syndrome (burning discomfort without signs of pathology)[2]

Xerostomia
- Related to the cancer itself (eg, head and neck cancer)
- Dehydration
- Radiotherapy
- Drug therapy (anticholinergic, psychotropic, opioid, cardiovascular, sympathetic agonist)[1]

Taste Disorders
- Sinusitis or other infections
- Xerostomia
- Medication side effects (eg, some antidepressants, HIV medications, chemotherapy)
- Vitamin or mineral deficiency (eg, zinc)[3]

Osteonecrosis of the Jaw
- Associated with the use of bisphosphonate medications; may occur following dental procedures (such as tooth extraction) or can occur spontaneously
- Was first described with the use of intravenous (IV) zolendronic acid and pamidronate, but also can occur with orally administered (PO) bisphosphonates (alendronate, risedronate, and ibandronate) commonly used for the treatment of osteoporosis[4]
- Common symptoms include facial or oral pain, soft tissue swelling, loosening of teeth, and drainage. Dental or oral surgical consultation should be considered for management.

Management of Oral Discomfort
Traumatic or aphthous lesions and oral mucositis from chemotherapy or radiation often heal in a couple of weeks. The patient's condition and goals of care should drive the intensity of involvement and evaluations from consultant groups. The use of consultant services, such as gastroenterology, otolaryngology, infectious disease, or oral surgery, in refractory cases often can provide further treatment recommendations. Many patients respond to nonspecific treatments, which are outlined below.

Dry Mouth/Xerostomia
- Minimize the use of anticholinergic medications whenever possible.
- Prescribe a saliva substitute, oral gel, or sugar-free chewing gum every 1 to 2 hours or as needed.[5]
- Prescribe 5 mg to 10 mg doses of PO pilocarpine three times per day (watch for increased respiratory secretions or diarrhea).[6]

- If possible, attempt to increase the patient's oral liquid intake by offering frozen juice, flavored ice, or popsicles. For patients unable or unwilling to take sufficient liquids, strategies can include eating ice chips, using an atomizer (eg, mist or spray), or frequently sipping water.
- As death approaches, encourage family members to keep the patient's mouth moist with a few drops of water from a syringe or a moist sponge stick. Lemon-flavored swabs or those containing glycerin may be irritating for some patients; generally a plain sponge and water is effective.
- The caregivers can keep a patient's lips moisturized with petroleum jelly or another nonirritating lip balm. These activities involve caregivers in the patient's care and may relieve dry mouth better than parenteral fluids.

Mucositis
- Chlorhexidine gluconate or oral lavage with 5 mL of sodium bicarbonate (baking soda) dissolved in water
- Combination mouthwash preparations containing two or three of the following:
  - diphenhydramine
  - topical lidocaine
  - nystatin
  - tetracycline
  - hydrocortisone
- Lidocaine 2%, 2 mL to 5 mL every 4 to 8 hours (can be diluted or flavored if desired; a 50/50 mixture with famotidine will allow for better adherence to tissues; can cause aspiration if used before meals)
- Sucralfate, 1 g/10 mL oral suspension, 5 mL to 10 mL swish and swallow three or four times daily
- Doxepin oral rinse, 25 mg/5 mL up to every 4 hours[7]
- Topical opioids (eg, dilute dose of scheduled opioid in water, swish and swallow, or spit)[8]
- Parenteral opioids

4B | Dysphagia

Swallowing difficulties are common at the end of life. They may be due to oropharyngeal problems, obstructing esophageal lesions (which often consists of difficulty first with swallowing solids and then tolerance for liquids only), esophageal dysmotility (neuromuscular or autoimmune etiology), or cognitive impairment. Dysphagia can be quite distressing to families, especially if patients develop a cough when attempting to take food, fluid, or medications orally.

Oropharyngeal Dysphagia

Some patients with oropharyngeal dysphagia may be assisted through simple interventions (eg, upright repositioning in bed, sitting at a table for meals), by changing the consistency of foods (ie, soft, pureed solids and thickened liquids), or with careful hand feeding by caregivers. Video-fluoroscopy and speech therapy consultation can be helpful for some patients who wish to continue eating without dietary modifications or the use of feeding tubes. The individual response to these types of interventions is variable, and diet consistency modifications may be unpalatable for many because they can adversely affect the pleasure patients experience from eating. Educating the family and caregivers is important to help them understand that swallowing difficulties are common toward the end of life and may not be due to any one specific reversible condition or disease process.

Esophageal Obstruction

The practitioner should also be alert to new symptoms suggesting esophageal spasm or obstruction (eg, recurrent chest pain, food sticking, regurgitation, vomiting). When dysphagia from esophageal obstruction is irreversible or progressive, the practitioner, interdisciplinary team, and patient and family should consider whether more invasive measures, such as the following, would be appropriate:

- surgical resection or laser ablation of an obstructing lesion
- placement of an esophageal stent[9]
- placement of a gastrostomy tube if hunger is present and ongoing nutrition is desired by the patient and family.

Helping the family cope with feelings of anxiety and guilt about the patient's low intake may be the most important intervention. Patients with dysphagia are at high risk for aspiration and aspiration pneumonia. Therefore, it is important to clarify goals of care regarding the future use of antibiotics should infection occur.

Hiccups

Hiccups (sometimes referred to as hiccoughs) can be an uncomfortable and distressing symptom for patients and their caregivers. Fortunately, most cases are acute, idiopathic, and self-limiting; however, chronic or intractable hiccups can interfere with eating and speaking, cause abdominal and chest pain, and adversely affect the overall quality of life for patients. Hiccups are caused by involuntary diaphragmatic muscular contractions that cause rapid inspiration and subsequently upper airway glottis closure, which produces the characteristic sound. Virtually any condition that causes diaphragmatic inflammation can be a precipitant of these myoclonic spasms, and many cases of hiccups are multifactorial. Malignancies involving the pleura, bowel, stomach, biliary tract, pancreas, or liver can cause diaphragmatic irritation. Past abdominal or thoracic surgeries also may be a risk factor. The clinician should be alert to the emergence of new hiccup symptoms that may indicate new clinical complications (such as infection, splenic infarction, electrolyte disturbances, or the development of renal failure) or be a sign of medication side effects or toxicity (such as from opioids, neuroleptics, and steroids).

Treatment of hiccups can involve both pharmacologic and nonpharmacologic interventions and there are many proposed folk remedies that have a limited evidence base (eg, breath holding, small sips of fluids, sweet or sour foods, acupuncture). The decision to use medications to treat hiccups should be individualized based on the chronicity, how bothersome the symptoms are to the patient, and the potential side effects of the chosen medication. A systematic review of hiccups in cancer patients found that a variety of medications have been used to treat these symptoms, including benzodiazepines, baclofen, gabapentin, chlorpromazine, methylphenidate, metoclopramide, amantadine, nifedipine, and haloperidol.[10] Many of these medications are available in both oral and parenteral routes of administration and have both peripheral and central nervous system modes of action. However, the use of these medications is mostly based on case reports and small case series with significant heterogeneity in both the patients and the medication dosages used. Some clinicians use a combination of medications to treat hiccups, but an additive increase in the side effects of the medications also needs to be considered.

4C | Artificial Nutrition and Hydration

Clinicians need to facilitate honest and thoughtful conversations with patients and their families regarding artificial nutrition and hydration (ANH). Clinicians may feel bound by legal and ethical obligations related to nutritional intake, and the family may have strong concerns about the perception that a loved one is "starving to death." Clinicians should try to understand and address the anxiety and fear associated with declining oral intake in patients approaching the end of life. Expectations and goals need to be clarified in these cases, and the relative benefits and limitations of ANH need to be discussed. The benefits from ANH for palliative care patients often are difficult to identify except under very particular circumstances (see below).

Feeding Tubes

Enteral nutrition can be given directly into the stomach by means of a nasogastric (NG) or percutaneous endoscopic gastrostomy (PEG) tube, thus bypassing the oral route for patients who have difficulty chewing and swallowing. PEG tubes were originally developed as a means of providing nutritional support for patients undergoing treatment for head and neck cancer, and their placement has generally been considered a safe procedure since first described in 1980.[11] The use of PEG tubes has markedly increased for a variety of other medical conditions, including advanced dementia, although research clearly indicates that PEG tubes are associated with considerable harm and do not provide a mortality benefit in such patients.[12-17] Decision making regarding feeding tubes is complex for individuals, often involving strong personal, family, or religious beliefs, and is complicated by misinformation (even within the medical community) regarding perceived and actual benefits.[18,19]

Tube feedings may be helpful for select patients, such as those with a tracheostomy or who require prolonged mechanical ventilation (if consistent with established goals of care), those with oropharyngeal or esophageal obstruction, or patients with neurologic disease affecting swallowing (eg, stroke or neurodegenerative disease such as amyotrophic lateral sclerosis).[20] The patients least likely to benefit from a feeding tube are those with a decline in oral intake due to progressive dementia or with weight loss and general debility due to overall declining health status and function (eg, "failure to thrive"). A major medical complication for patients with swallowing problems is the development of aspiration pneumonia. Aspiration risk is increased for patients with dysphagia, but evidence indicates that there is no significant reduction in aspiration events with the placement of a PEG tube.[12,21]

Patients with dementia may pull on NG or PEG tubes, leading hospital or nursing home staff to put physical restraints in place, thereby exacerbating suffering, delirium, or agitation. Feeding tubes can become obstructed or dislodged, and infection or bleeding can develop around the percutaneous tract (requiring hospital transfers for interventions and tube replacement), all of which potentially may add to the burden of the feeding tube. In light of the limited benefits and considerable burdens of feeding tubes, clinicians should explore alternative ways to meet nutritional goals, such as a careful hand-feeding program (see **Table 4.1**).

Total Parenteral Nutrition

The evidence for ANH for patients with cancer is heterogeneous, reflecting the nature of the cancer population, and includes differences in cancer types and trajectories of disease progression. Total parenteral nutrition (TPN) for cancer patients rarely is beneficial because of metabolic derangements characteristic of the cachexia syndrome.[21,22] Select patients, such as postsurgical oncology patients who are unable to tolerate enteral nutrition (eg, due to bowel obstruction or prolonged ileus) but are expected to recover bowel function over time, could benefit

Table 4.1 Benefits and Burdens of PEG Placement

	Dysphagic Stroke (Patients with previously good quality of life, high functional status,[1] and minimal comorbidities)	Dysphagic Stroke (Patients with decreased level of consciousness, multiple co-morbidities, and poor functional status[1] prior to cerebrovascular accident)	Amyotrophic Lateral Sclerosis (ALS or Lou Gehrig's Disease)	Persistent Vegetative State (PVS)	General Frailty (Patients with multiple comorbidities, poor functional status, and failure to thrive)	Advanced Dementia (Patients needing help with daily care, having trouble communicating, or experiencing incontinence)	Advanced Cancer (Excludes patients with early-stage esophageal and oral cancer)	Advanced Organ Failure (Patients with congestive heart failure, renal or liver failure, chronic obstructive pulmonary disease, or anorexia-cachexia)
Prolongs Life	Likely	Likely in the short term / Not likely in the long term	Likely	Likely	Not Likely	Not Likely[2]	Not Likely	Not Likely
Improves Quality of Life and/or Functional Status	Up to 25% regain swallowing capabilities	Not likely	Uncertain	Not Likely	Not Likely	Not Likely	Not Likely	Not Likely
Enables Potentially Curative Therapy/Reverses the Disease	Not Likely	Not Likely	Not Likely	Not Likely	Not Likely	Not Likely	Not Likely	Not Likely

Benefits of PEG placement rather than feeding orally

- For dysphagic stroke patients previously in good health, patients with ALS, and patients in a PVS, may prolong life
- For dysphagic stroke patients previously in poor health, may prolong life in the short term (days to weeks)
- Enables family members and caregivers to maintain hope for future improvement
- Enables family members and caregivers to avoid guilt or conflict associated with choosing other treatment options
- Allows family members and caregivers additional time to adjust to the possibility of impending death

Burdens of PEG placement rather than feeding orally

- Seventy-five percent of stroke patients previously in good health are not likely to have improved quality of life or functional status.
- PVS patients are not likely to have improved quality of life or functional status.
- Possible patient agitation resulting in use of restraints
- Risk of aspiration pneumonia is the same or greater than that of a patient being handfed
- Stroke patients previously in poor health; frail patients; and patients with advanced dementia, cancer, or organ failure have been reported to experience side effects: PEG site irritation or leaking (21%), diarrhea (22%), nausea (13%), and vomiting (20%).[3]

Benefits of feeding orally rather than inserting a PEG

- Patient is able to enjoy the taste of food
- Patient has greater opportunity for social interaction
- Patient's wishes and circumstances can be taken into consideration in terms of pacing, timing, and volume of feeding

Burdens of feeding orally rather than inserting a PEG

- Requires longer period of time to feed a patient
- Patient and family worry about "not doing everything in their power" to address the feeding problem or "starving the patient"
- Patient and family feel that in not choosing an option that possibly could prolong life, they are hastening death

This information is based predominately on a consensus of current expert opinion. It is not exhaustive. There are always patients who prove exceptions to the rule.

1. Functional status refers to activities of daily living. A poor functional status means full or partial dependency in bathing, dressing, toileting, feeding, ambulation, or transfers.

2. There is a small group of patients who fall into this category whose lives could be prolonged.

3. Callahan CM, Haag KM, Weinberger M, et al. Outcomes of percutaneous endoscopic gastrostomy among older adults in a community setting. *J Am Geriatr Soc.* 2000 Sep; 48(9):1048-1054.

Monroe County Medical Society. Rochester Community-Wide Practice Guidelines: Tube Feeding/PEGs. Monroe County Medical Society Quality Collaborative website. http://cwcg.mcms.org/CWCGClinicalGuidelines.aspx. *Accessed September 15, 2013.*

from TPN. It also is important to consider the high cost and significant, potentially adverse effects of TPN, including infections, liver failure, or thrombosis.

Intravenous Hydration

The administration of IV fluids rarely reverses circulatory shutdown at the end stages of illness and potentially can cause fluid overload, particularly as renal function decreases. Parenteral hydration did not improve symptoms, survival, or quality of life in a randomized trial of patients with advanced cancer.[23] Therefore, clinicians need to educate patients and families about the increased risk of third-space fluid retention and respiratory congestion. Others have suggested that a short-term trial of parenteral hydration via IV or subcutaneous (SC) routes (ie, hypodermoclysis) may be worthwhile to help mitigate mental status changes, generalized weakness, or malaise in patients with an anticipated life expectancy of at least several days.[24] Hypodermoclysis has proven to be practical in this population and offers the advantage of avoiding the need to establish peripheral IV access.[25]

Discussions with Patients and Families

Most clinicians familiar with end-of-life care report that patients do not experience hunger or thirst at this time, do not request food or fluid beyond a taste or mouth moistening, and remain comfortable and peaceful as long as other symptoms are aggressively controlled. Death occurs because of the underlying illness, not because of the lack of food or fluids. Despite this, clinicians need to be observant of cultural and spiritual sensitivities that may influence a patient's or family's insistence on the continuation of ANH, even when there may be little or no medical benefit in continuing the intervention.

If ANH is being considered, the clinician, interdisciplinary team, patient, and family need to establish a time frame to evaluate whether predetermined goals have been achieved. For example, if weight loss or overall decline continues despite ANH, the clinician can recommend its cessation. The development of complications with ANH (eg, swelling, skin breakdown, infection at the infusion site) also might lead to the discontinuation of interventions. Clinicians need to educate families that a lack of nutrition and fluids does not increase the suffering of dying patients; in fact, decreased intake is a normal part of the dying process.

The clinician should involve an interdisciplinary team, including a chaplain or other spiritual advisor appropriate for the patient, in periodic discussions about goals of care and whether ANH therapy continues to meet those goals. For example, the team and family may agree to decrease the rate of tube feedings when there is evidence of respiratory congestion near the end of life or discontinue these feedings when there is obvious dyspnea, vomiting, or aspiration.

Alternative Routes of Medication Administration

Oral Concentrates

Several medications can be given as oral concentrates, including opioids (morphine and oxycodone concentrated solutions are both available at 20 mg/mL) and sedatives/antiemetics (haloperidol and lorazepam are available at 2 mg/mL). If patients are able to swallow their oral secretions and are not actively vomiting, they may be able to ingest these medications because of their small volumes.

Transcutaneous Preparations

Fentanyl and scopolamine are readily available in transcutaneous preparations. Other medications can be compounded by some pharmacies, although the reliability of absorption remains unproven.

Subcutaneous Bolus Doses or Infusions

When central or IV lines are in place, they may be used to administer parenteral medications. Inserting new catheters will depend on a patient's clinical circumstances and the goals of treatment. If treatment is purely palliative and parenteral administration is needed (when less invasive routes are ineffective), consider using SC bolus doses or infusions.[26] Most families can be taught to give injections into an injection site or through an SC butterfly needle. The volume of drug given should be less than 1.5 mL per injection to avoid discomfort.

Alternatively, a solution bag or simple pump can be used to deliver a continuous infusion of SC medications.[27] Many antiemetic medications can be given by continuous SC infusion through a 21- to 25-gauge butterfly needle, usually up to a maximum rate of 1 mL to 2 mL per hour. The injection site can be changed every 2 to 7 days but the exact interval for rotating to a new site should be based upon clinical judgment, including observations of any erythema, swelling, or discomfort at the infusion site.[28]

Rectal Suppositories

Many antiemetic agents may be delivered using custom-made rectal (PR) suppositories (eg, chlorpromazine suppositories may be given in 25 mg to 100 mg doses every 4 to 8 hours). Some slow-release analgesic tablets can also be administered rectally.[29,30] However, PR administration may be limited by patient modesty, the lack of availability of custom-made suppositories, overflow diarrhea, and the discomfort and embarrassment of rectally administering multiple drugs on a scheduled basis.

4D | Nausea and Vomiting

Nausea and vomiting are some of the most distressing symptoms in palliative care. They occur in up to 20% to 30% of all patients with advanced cancer and are most common in those with advanced gynecological and gastrointestinal (GI) cancer (up to 40% to 50%). They also occur in other advanced illnesses, including end-stage cardiac, renal, and liver disease. Protracted nausea and vomiting can affect appetite, pain management, and the quality of interactions with family or friends, and can make life simply miserable.

The pathophysiology of vomiting (**Figure 4.1**) is better understood than that of many other symptoms. A section of the midbrain, the vomiting center, coordinates the vomiting reflex and receives input from various sources.

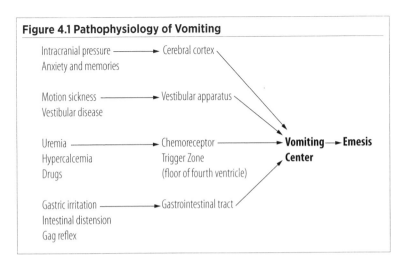

Figure 4.1 Pathophysiology of Vomiting

Intracranial pressure ⟶ Cerebral cortex
Anxiety and memories

Motion sickness ⟶ Vestibular apparatus
Vestibular disease

Uremia ⟶ Chemoreceptor ⟶ **Vomiting** ⟶ **Emesis**
Hypercalcemia Trigger Zone **Center**
Drugs (floor of fourth ventricle)

Gastric irritation ⟶ Gastrointestinal tract
Intestinal distension
Gag reflex

Patient Assessment

History and Examination

A focused history should include the type of advanced illness, the stage of illness, relationship with meals, relationship with head motion, the extent and type of vomiting, changes in bowel patterns, the presence or absence of other GI-related or neurological symptoms, and a thorough review of medications. Given the broad differential diagnosis, a thorough physical exam is needed but should be focused on the GI (eg, oral mucosa, bowel sounds, ascites, rectum) and components of the neurological exam (eg, papilledema, presence of nystagmus, mental status changes, focal findings).

Diagnostic Work-Up

The diagnostic work-up will depend in part on the stage of the illness and the goals of care. The workup may include blood draws for chemistry (calcium, sodium, blood urea nitrogen [BUN], bilirubin) and drug levels (theophylline, digoxin, antiepileptic drugs). Neuroradiologic imaging may be needed to rule out potential sources of increased intracranial pressure or unusual brainstem causes of vertigo and nausea. If an intra-abdominal source is considered, an abdominal image (X ray, ultrasound, or computed tomography) may be indicated.

Etiology-Specific Causes of Nausea and Vomiting

When evaluating and managing patients with nausea and vomiting, consider whether the symptoms are being caused by intra-abdominal factors (eg, gastroparesis, ileus, gastric outlet obstruction, bowel obstruction) or extra-abdominal factors (eg, drugs, electrolyte abnormalities, central nervous system [CNS] metastases). In palliative care, intra-abdominal causes are more likely and often present with an obstructive component. The goal is to identify and treat underlying reversible causes, but the practical reality is that empiric pharmacologic treatment is usually needed to immediately control symptoms. Table 4.2 provides etiology-specific causes of nausea and vomiting in the palliative care setting.

Table 4.2 Causes and Treatment for Nausea and Vomiting in Palliative Care

SPECIFIC CAUSE	LOOK FOR	CONSIDER
Gastrointestinal Tract		
Bowel inflammation or compression (eg, tumor infiltration, ascites, hepatosplenomegaly, radiation therapy to the GI tract, or infection)	*Candida esophagitis*, colitis, massive abdominal distension, gastric compression, history of radiation therapy	Haloperidol: Start at 0.5 mg SC or 1 mg PO every 6-12 hours; increase up to 5 mg-20 mg per day in divided doses[31,32]
		Consider higher dose PO/IV/SC metoclopramide 60 mg-240 mg per day or PO/SL olanzapine 5-10 mg daily[33,34]
Bowel obstruction or poor motility	Constipation unrelieved by treatment, abdominal colic, response to motility agent	See Table 4.3 for pharmacologic options for bowel obstruction.
Irritation by drugs	Use of NSAIDs, iron, alcohol, antibiotics	Stop drug if possible; add proton pump inhibitor, H2 blocker, or misoprostol

Table 4.2 Causes and Treatment for Nausea and Vomiting in Palliative Care *continued*

SPECIFIC CAUSE	LOOK FOR	CONSIDER
Constipation or impaction	Abdominal distension, extended time since last bowel movement, impaction on rectal exam	Laxative (see detailed recommendations later in this chapter), manual disimpaction, or enema prn
Tube feedings	Abdominal distension, diarrhea	Reduce volume or stop feeding; change from bolus feeding to continuous
Nasopharyngeal bleeding	Hemoptysis, epistaxis, blood visible in pharynx	Nasal packing, vitamin K if appropriate, sedation
Thick respiratory secretions	Cough-induced vomiting (post-tussive emesis)	Nebulized saline; expectorant if good cough reflex, anticholinergic if poor cough reflex
Chemoreceptor Trigger Zone[†]		
Drugs (eg, opiates, chemotherapy, digoxin, carbamazepine, phenytoin, antibiotics, theophylline)	Nausea worse after drug started; exacerbated by increased drug dosage	Decrease drug dosage or discontinue drug, if possible
Metabolic (eg, renal or liver failure or tumor products)	Increased BUN, creatinine, bilirubin	Biliary or ureteral stint if appropriate
		Haloperidol: Start at 0.5 mg SC or 1.0 mg PO every 6 hours or every 12 hours; increase up to 5 mg-20 mg per day in divided doses[31,32]
		Olanzapine 2.5 mg-10 mg PO/SL at bedtime[33]
Hyponatremia	Confusion, low sodium	Salt tablets or demeclocycline
Hypercalcemia	Somnolence, delirium, high calcium	Hydration and pamidronate 60 mg-90 mg IV or zoledronic acid 4mg IV

continued

Table 4.2 Causes and Treatment for Nausea and Vomiting in Palliative Care *continued*

SPECIFIC CAUSE	LOOK FOR	CONSIDER
Cortical		
Tumor in CNS or meninges	Neurologic signs or mental status problems	Dexamethasone 4 mg-8 mg PO/SC/IV every 4-8 hours; consider radiation therapy for new metastases
Increased intracranial pressure	Projectile vomiting, headache	Dexamethasone 4 mg-8 mg PO/SC/IV every 4-8 hours
Anxiety and other conditioned responses	Anticipatory nausea, predictable vomiting	Counseling; benzodiazepines (eg, lorazepam): 0.5 mg-1.5 mg PO/SC/IV every 4-8 hours
Uncontrolled pain	Pain and nausea	Opiates, other pain medications, and adjuvants
Vestibular/Middle Ear		
Vestibular disease	Vertigo or vomiting after head motion	Meclizine or hydroxyzine: 25 mg PO three times daily or transdermal scopolamine; consider ENT consult
Middle ear infections	Ear pain or bulging tympanic membrane	Antibiotic and decongestant, as appropriate
Motion sickness	Travel-related nausea	TD scopolamine, meclizine, or hydroxyzine 25 mg PO three times daily

BUN, blood urea nitrogen; ENT, otolaryngology (ear, nose, and throat); NSAIDs, nonsteroidal anti-inflammatory drugs; PO, oral; prn, as needed; SC, subcutaneous; SL, sublingual; TD, transdermal; IV, intravenous.

†*This is the area of the brain that senses changes in the blood and mediates most common causes of nausea.*

Pharmacologic Management

Scheduling regular doses of antiemetics often can prevent recurrent nausea. If the patient is too nauseated to tolerate oral medications, consider SC, IV, or PR routes. High dosages of a combination of agents may be required. One of the most useful medications to treat nausea in palliative care is haloperidol.[32] Like other antipsychotics, haloperidol now carries a black box warning from the US Food and Drug Administration (FDA) regarding an increased risk of mortality in patients with dementia. An initial dose of haloperidol, 1 mg PO (or PR) or 0.5 mg SC (or IV) two to three times daily, is recommended to relieve nausea; however, this dosage may need to be increased to up to 20 mg per day.[31,32,35] Extrapyramidal side effects are much less of a concern over a short duration of use or with limited life expectancy. For patients with existing Parkinsonian symptoms, a moderate to high dosage of olanzapine may be effective for nausea,[33,34] but it is expensive, has the same FDA black box warning as haloperidol, and can worsen motor symptoms.

Depending on the potential etiology, additional medications may be indicated. For example, when nausea and vomiting are due to increased intracranial pressure, a steroid such as dexamethasone (4 mg PO, SC, IV, or PR two to four times daily) is useful. In situations of delayed gastric emptying or early satiety, metoclopramide (5 mg to 20 mg PO, SC, or IV three to four times daily) may be useful. Although 5-HT$_3$ serotonin receptor antagonists such as ondansetron, granisetron, or dolasetron and NK$_1$ antagonists such as aprepitant are effective in alleviating chemotherapy-induced nausea, they may not be as useful for managing nausea and vomiting in advanced illness.[36] When an anxiety component exists (particularly in cases of anticipatory nausea with medications or food), lorazepam (0.5 mg to 1 mg PO, SC, or IV three times daily) can be helpful in reducing anxiety symptoms. When nausea and vomiting are due to inner-ear pathology or motion sickness, antihistamines such as hydroxyzine (25 mg to 50 mg PO, IV, PR, or SC [watch for SC irritation] two to four times daily) can help manage vertigo. Promethazine and meclizine are additional options, but often patients find these medications sedating. For intractable nausea and vomiting, octreotide 100 mcg to 600 mcg SC or IV two or three times daily has demonstrated some benefit, particularly in bowel obstruction.[37-39]

If nausea is refractory despite adequate dosing and around-the-clock prophylactic administration, management strategies should focus on empirical trials combining several medications that target multiple emetic pathways.[40] A venting gastrostomy may also be considered in extreme cases.

Management of Nausea and Vomiting with Bowel Obstruction

When patients with terminal illness develop bowel obstructions, the therapeutic goal is to manage the symptoms (eg, no pain, no cramps, minimal nausea, no more than one emesis per day) and to maximize quality of life.[41] Most bowel obstructions are partial obstructions and can be managed effectively with medications (**Table 4.3**). When symptoms are controlled, quality of life improves, not only because symptom relief has been achieved but also because patients may be able to drink fluids and eat small amounts of their favorite foods.

Surgical intervention, venting gastrostomy, or metallic stenting can be useful in some patients with advanced gynecologic or GI cancers and should be considered as part of the palliative management plan.[42,43] For instance, a venting gastrostomy may be helpful for high-grade proximal obstructions because NG suction and IV fluids for symptom control are uncomfortable and rarely are necessary or helpful for long-term use. Surgical interventions may not be practical because of patient debility or multiple sites of obstruction.

Successful symptom control often can be achieved by using a combination of analgesic, anticholinergic, and antiemetic drugs.[41,44] The route of drug administration must be individualized; medication dosages and combinations will require frequent readjustment. Multiple antiemetics often will need to be tried (see Table 4.2). For intractable symptoms and in the setting of a partial obstruction, combinations of an opioid, dexamethasone, haloperidol, metoclopramide, and octreotide may be needed via a parenteral route. Non-drug methods such as guided imagery or acupuncture also should be considered.[45] Patience, persistence, and reassurance are needed by the provider, patient, and caregiver while achieving symptom control.

Patient and Caregiver Education

Involve all members of the team to help treat the social, psychological, and spiritual aspects of nausea and vomiting. Several general treatment measures directed at caregivers and patients should be encouraged.

Patient
- Get enough rest.
- Avoid disagreeable foods and odors.
- Avoid fatty and fried foods.
- Try a mint or other hard candy for disagreeable tastes in the mouth.
- Take most medications, except antiemetics, after eating.

Caregivers
- Provide small, frequent meals consisting of foods chosen by the patient.
- Provide liquids frequently.
- Provide a quiet, relaxing, and pleasant atmosphere.
- Provide companionship for meals.
- Teach the patient relaxation techniques.

Table 4.3 Pharmacologic Options for Bowel Obstruction		
DRUG	**DOSAGE**	**COMMENT**
Pain		
Morphine or hydromorphone	Titrate to relief PO/SL/SC/IV (remember, morphine SC dose = 1/3 PO dose and hydromorphone SC dose = 1/5 PO dose)	For cramping pain (colic), may need high dosage or addition of glycopyrrolate or hyoscyamine; if pain is unrelieved, consider celiac plexus block
Nausea		
Haloperidol	5 mg-20 mg/day PO/SC/IV (haloperidol 2 mg PO route is equivalent to 1 mg SC/IV routes)	Mix in 5% dextrose for SC infusion; inexpensive

continued

Table 4.3 Pharmacologic Options for Bowel Obstruction *continued*

DRUG	DOSAGE	COMMENT
Metoclopramide	60 mg-240 mg/day SC/PO/IV	May cause colic if opioid dosage is low; may be effective in partial obstructions or ileus; can worsen Parkinsonian motor symptoms; may aggravate cramping in complete obstruction
Chlorpromazine	25 mg-100 mg/tid PO/PR/IV	Useful if some of the above agents are unavailable; can be sedating; irritating if administered SC, use other administration routes
Persistent Vomiting		
Dexamethasone	Start at 4 mg PO/SC/IV two to four times daily	May relieve malignant bowel obstruction[46]
Transdermal scopolamine	1-3 patches topically behind ear; change every 72 hours	Slows gut; can cause dry mouth, blurred vision
Glycopyrrolate	0.4 mg every 4 hours SC bolus or by 0.2 mg-1.0 mg/day SC infusion[47]	Slows gut; can cause dry mouth, urinary retention, confusion
Hyoscyamine	0.125 mg SL every 4-8 hours	Slows gut; can cause dry mouth, urinary retention, confusion
Octreotide	Start 50 mcg-200 mcg SC three times daily or continuous SC infusion starting at 10 mcg-20 mcg/hour	Reduces intestinal secretions and slows gut; may be useful in acute management of bowel obstruction[37-39]; requires injections or infusion and is expensive

IV, intravenous; PO, oral; PR, rectal; SC, subcutaneous; SL, sublingual; tid, three times daily.

4E | Constipation

The principal challenges to managing this distressing symptom are vigilant prevention and early recognition and treatment if it occurs. Legend has it that Cicely Saunders once gave an hour-long lecture in which every fourth slide read, "Nothing matters more than the bowels!"

Constipation is prevalent in end-of-life care and involves a complex interaction of anatomic, neurologic, and iatrogenic factors.[48] Palliative medicine patients are at high risk due to the following factors:

- low intake of food, fluid, and fiber
- impaired mobility
- opioid analgesics and other drugs that impair gut motility
- complicating medical conditions, such as bowel obstruction or hemorrhoids.

A careful assessment includes a directed history (including stool frequency, consistency, laxative use, and associated problems, such as lack of privacy or a long distance to the toilet), an abdominal examination, and a rectal examination. If a hard fecal impaction is found, soften it with an oil retention enema. The patient then should receive sedating medication (eg, lorazepam, midazolam) before the impaction is removed digitally. Soft impaction may respond to bisacodyl suppositories or large-volume saline enemas. This should be followed by a vigorous program involving both a stool softener and a stimulant agent (eg, senna, bisacodyl) to prevent recurrence. Patients with recurrent or severe constipation should be monitored daily.[49]

Many patients require a maintenance bowel regimen to prevent or relieve constipation. Patients who are started on regular doses of an opioid analgesic should receive a regularly scheduled laxative, and most will benefit from a combination of a stool softener and a stimulant.[50] The treatment of constipation in palliative care is based on limited research evidence, and most patients will require both a scheduled medication regimen and the use of rescue medications for episodes of constipation.[50,51] In general, bulk-forming fiber agents (eg, psyllium, methylcellulose) have little role in palliative care because of their tendency to form impactions when patients stop taking in adequate amounts of fluids. If a patient has a history of constipation, use the patient's preferred home regimen before starting new medications. Medications can be added in a stepwise fashion; however, increasing the dosage or frequency of existing bowel medications usually is effective. Table 4.4 lists various types of medications and dosing.

Table 4.4 Prevention and Treatment of Constipation

MEDICATION	DOSAGE AND FREQUENCY	COMMENTS
Stool Softener (Detergent Laxative)		
Docusate sodium (capsules/tablets or liquid)	Starting dose: 100 mg PO twice daily or 200 mg; titrate dose up to two or three times daily. Max. 600 mg daily	Generally well tolerated and safe; generally insufficient if used alone[52]
Stimulants		
Senna	1 tab PO daily; titrate up to 4 tabs PO twice daily	Useful when added to docusate; can worsen colic in bowel obstruction
Bisacodyl	Start with 1 (5 mg) tab PO daily; titrate to 3 tabs twice daily. Suppository 10 mg PR daily prn	Can worsen colic in bowel obstruction; bisacodyl suppository causes more cramping than glycerin suppository; bisacodyl tablets can cause more cramping than senna tablets
Osmotic Agents		
Glycerin suppository	1 PR daily prn	Acts as both lubricant and osmotic agent; generally well tolerated, but rarely adequate alone
Sorbitol	15 mL–60 mL PO two to four times daily	Sweet taste can be unpleasant; can cause bloating
Lactulose (10 g/ 15 mL)	15 mL–60 mL PO two or three times daily	More expensive than sorbitol but with similar efficacy and side effects[53]
Polyethylene glycol	17 g powder dissolved in liquid PO one to three times daily	Tasteless; often well tolerated; available over the counter
Milk of Magnesia	15 mL–30 mL daily prn	Can cause cramping; high magnesium load with renal failure
Magnesium citrate	1–2 bottles prn	Can cause cramping; high magnesium load with renal failure

Table 4.4 Prevention and Treatment of Constipation continued

MEDICATION	DOSAGE AND FREQUENCY	COMMENTS
Enemas		
Warm "tap" water	One PR administration, can repeat daily or twice daily	PR administration can soften stool before manual disimpaction
Saline or sodium phosphate	One PR administration	**USE IS NOT RECOMMENDED:** There is a high electrolyte load, which may cause dehydration, renal failure, or exacerbation of hepatic or cardiac failure in some patients. Risk is highest in pediatric and older adult patients
Mineral oil	One PR administration	Oral dosing should be avoided; risk of severe pneumonitis if aspirated; PR administration can soften stool before manual disimpaction
Milk and molasses (or corn syrup)	Added to a liter of water; PR administration	Combines both osmotic and colonic stimulant; traditional use has been when all else fails
Soap suds	One PR administration	Not recommended: colon irritant, risk of bowel-wall damage with large dose or repeated use
Other Agents		
Prune juice	120 mL–240 mL PO one or two times daily	Combines both soluble fiber and stimulant; a recognized traditional approach; good adjuvant
Metoclopramide	10 mg–20 mg PO every 6 hours	Promotility agent; may be helpful for some patients; contraindicated in complete bowel obstruction; potential for tardive dyskinesia (FDA black box warning); avoid prolonged use
Methylnaltrexone	0.15 mg/kg of body weight (up to 12 mg) SC injection every other day	Need to rule out bowel obstruction prior to administration; requires SC injection; usually produces bowel movement within 30 minutes; peripheral mu-opioid receptor antagonist; effectively treats opioid-induced constipation without reversing analgesia or precipitating withdrawal[54-56]; expensive, generally used as rescue therapy in refractory cases
Lubiprostone	8 mcg–24 mcg PO twice daily with food	Chloride channel activator; FDA approved for constipation-predominant irritable bowel syndrome and chronic idiopathic constipation; may cause nausea[54,57]

FDA, US Food and Drug Administration; PO, oral; PR, rectal; prn, as needed; SC, subcutaneous.

If constipation has never been a problem, docusate or docusate plus senna may be an initial starting point. However, the efficacy of docusate alone is limited, and most patients will require a bowel stimulant like senna or bisacodyl in substantial doses (increasing up to four tablets twice daily). Tolerance to stimulant laxatives is uncommon. Bowel obstructions may be a contraindication to stimulant laxatives because they may increase colic. Colicky abdominal pains can be minimized with careful dose titration and the addition of docusate for stool softening. Patients who are still passing some stool through obstructions can benefit from a softening agent such as higher-dose docusate or an osmotic agent such as sorbitol or polyethylene glycol.

Osmotic agents (such as sorbitol 70% or lactulose 10 g/15 mL concentrations) are effective additions to most bowel regimens (eg, give 15 mL to 60 mL two or three times daily), especially if stimulants alone are ineffective or poorly tolerated. Bloating, flatulence, dislike of the sickly sweet taste, and diarrhea can be problematic. Sorbitol is less expensive, equally effective, and less nauseating than lactulose.[53] Polyethylene glycol is tasteless, odorless, and generally well tolerated by patients. It has been found effective for opioid induced constipation and there is evidence that it may be more effective than lactulose for chronic constipation.[58,59]

If constipation is severe, some patients may prefer a purgative dose of an oral osmotic agent prior to the use of an enema; however, cramping and nausea may be side effects. Rectal suppositories and enemas can be used when constipation is severe, but following the previously outlined management recommendations should minimize their use as part of a bowel regimen. In cases of bowel obstruction, consider constipation as an underlying cause or contributing factor in high-risk patients.

Further Discussion

1. How would you explain to patients and families the potential benefits and burdens of using a percutaneous endoscopic gastrostomy tube?

2. What are some strategies to treat dry mouth?

3. For patients with bowel obstruction due to cancer, what treatment options can be offered?

4. What is an appropriate starting medication regimen to prevent opioid-related constipation?

5. What is the role of fiber supplementation in opioid-related constipation?

6. What are the indications, methods of action, and limitations for using methylnaltrexone to treat opioid-related constipation?

7. What are the major locations in the body that may trigger nausea?

8. What are some medication strategies to manage intractable hiccups?

9. What are some alternative routes/methods for administering medications when a patient is unable to swallow?

10. What are the safety risks of using saline or sodium phosphate enemas in patients?

References

1. Epstein JB. Mucositis in the cancer patient and immunosuppressed host. *Infect Dis Clin North Am.* 2007;21(2):503-522, vii.

2. Klasser GD, Fischer DJ, Epstein JB. Burning mouth syndrome: recognition, understanding, and management. *Oral Maxillofac Surg Clin North Am.* 2008;20(2):255-271.

3. Halyard MY, Jatoi A, Sloan JA, et al. Does zinc sulfate prevent therapy-induced taste alterations in head and neck cancer patients? Results of

phase III double-blind, placebo-controlled trial from the North Central Cancer Treatment Group (N01C4). *Int J Radiat Oncol Biol Phys.* 2007;67(5):1318-1322.

4. Woo SB, Hande K, Richardson PG. Osteonecrosis of the jaw and bisphosphonates. *N Engl J Med.* 2005;353(1):99-102.

5. Davies AN. A comparison of artificial saliva and chewing gum in the management of xerostomia in patients with advanced cancer. *Palliat Med.* 2000;14(3):197-203.

6. Davies AN, Shorthose K. Parasympathomimetic drugs for the treatment of salivary gland dysfunction due to radiotherapy. *Cochrane Database Syst Rev.* 2007(3):CD003782.

7. Epstein JB, Epstein JD, Epstein MS, Oien H, Truelove EL. Oral doxepin rinse: the analgesic effect and duration of pain reduction in patients with oral mucositis due to cancer therapy. *Anesth Analg.* 2006;103(2):465-470.

8. Gairard-Dory AC, Schaller C, Mennecier B, et al. Chemoradiotherapy-induced esophagitis pain relieved by topical morphine: three cases. *J Pain Symptom Manage.* 2005;30(2):107-109.

9. Papachristou GI, Baron TH. Use of stents in benign and malignant esophageal disease. *Rev Gastroenterol Disord.* 2007;7(2):74-88.

10. Calsina-Berna A, Garcia-Gomez G, Gonzalez-Barboteo J, Porta-Sales J. Treatment of chronic hiccups in cancer patients: a systematic review. *J Palliat Med.* 2012;15(10):1142-1150.

11. Gauderer MW, Ponsky JL, Izant RJ, Jr. Gastrostomy without laparotomy: a percutaneous endoscopic technique. *J Pediatr Surg.* 1980;15(6):872-875.

12. Finucane TE, Christmas C, Travis K. Tube feeding in patients with advanced dementia: a review of the evidence. *JAMA.* 1999;282(14):1365-1370.

13. Barrocas A, Geppert C, Durfee SM, et al. A.S.P.E.N. ethics position paper. *Nutr Clin Pract.* 2010;25(6):672-679.

14. Teno JM, Gozalo P, Mitchell SL, Kuo S, Fulton AT, Mor V. Feeding tubes and the prevention or healing of pressure ulcers. *Arch Intern Med.* 2012;172(9):697-701.

15. Sampson EL, Candy B, Jones L. Enteral tube feeding for older people with advanced dementia. *Cochrane Database Syst Rev.* 2009(2):CD007209.

16. Meier DE, Ahronheim JC, Morris J, Baskin-Lyons S, Morrison RS. High short-term mortality in hospitalized patients with advanced dementia: lack of benefit of tube feeding. *Arch Intern Med.* 2001;161(4):594-599.

17. Mitchell SL, Kiely DK, Lipsitz LA. The risk factors and impact on survival of feeding tube placement in nursing home residents with severe cognitive impairment. *Arch Intern Med.* 1997;157(3):327-332.

18. Mitchell SL, Berkowitz RE, Lawson FM, Lipsitz LA. A cross-national survey of tube-feeding decisions in cognitively impaired older persons. *J Am Geriatr Soc.* 2000;48(4):391-397.

19. Orrevall Y, Tishelman C, Permert J, Lundstrom S. A national observational study of the prevalence and use of enteral tube feeding, parenteral nutrition and intravenous glucose in cancer patients enrolled in specialized palliative care. *Nutrients.* 2013;5(1):267-282.

20. Braun MM, Osecheck M, Joyce NC. Nutrition assessment and management in amyotrophic lateral sclerosis. *Phys Med Rehabil Clin N Am.* 2012;23(4):751-771.

21. Finucane TE, Bynum JP. Use of tube feeding to prevent aspiration pneumonia. *Lancet.* 1996;348(9039):1421-1424.

22. Bozzetti F, Arends J, Lundholm K, Micklewright A, Zurcher G, Muscaritoli M. ESPEN Guidelines on Parenteral Nutrition: non-surgical oncology. *Clin Nutr.* 2009;28(4):445-454.

23. Bruera E, Hui D, Dalal S, et al. Parenteral hydration in patients with advanced cancer: a multicenter, double-blind, placebo-controlled randomized trial. *J Clin Oncol.* 2013;31(1):111-118.

24. Lanuke K, Fainsinger RL, DeMoissac D. Hydration management at the end of life. *J Palliat Med.* 2004;7(2):257-263.

25. Lybarger EH. Hypodermoclysis in the home and long-term care settings. *J Infus Nurs.* 2009;32(1):40-44.

26. Parsons HA, Shukkoor A, Quan H, et al. Intermittent subcutaneous opioids for the management of cancer pain. *J Palliat Med.* 2008;11(10):1319-1324.

27. Menahem S, Shvartzman P. Continuous subcutaneous delivery of medications for home care palliative patients-using an infusion set or a pump? *Support Care Cancer.* 2010;18(9):1165-1170.

28. Mitchell K, Pickard J, Herbert A, Lightfoot J, Roberts D. Incidence and causes for syringe driver site reactions in palliative care: a prospective hospice-based study. *Palliat Med.* 2012;26(8):979-985.

29. Wilkinson TJ, Robinson BA, Begg EJ, Duffull SB, Ravenscroft PJ, Schneider JJ. Pharmacokinetics and efficacy of rectal versus oral sustained-release morphine in cancer patients. *Cancer Chemother Pharmacol.* 1992;31(3):251-254.

30. Walsh D, Tropiano PS. Long-term rectal administration of high-dose sustained-release morphine tablets. *Support Care Cancer.* 2002;10(8):653-655.

31. McLean SL, Blenkinsopp A, Bennett MI. Using haloperidol as an antiemetic in palliative care: informing practice through evidence from cancer treatment and postoperative contexts. *J Pain Palliat Care Pharmacother.* 2013;27(2):132-135.

32. Hardy JR, O'Shea A, White C, Gilshenan K, Welch L, Douglas C. The efficacy of haloperidol in the management of nausea and vomiting in patients with cancer. *J Pain Symptom Manage.* 2010;40(1):111-116.

33. Navari RM, Nagy CK, Gray SE. The use of olanzapine versus metoclopramide for the treatment of breakthrough chemotherapy-induced nausea and vomiting in patients receiving highly emetogenic chemotherapy. *Support Care Cancer.* 2013;21(6):1655-1663.

34. Mizukami N, Yamauchi M, Koike K, et al. Olanzapine for the prevention of chemotherapy-induced nausea and vomiting in patients receiving highly or moderately emetogenic chemotherapy: a randomized, double-blind, placebo-controlled study. *J Pain Symptom Manage.* 2013.

35. Critchley P, Plach N, Grantham M, et al. Efficacy of haloperidol in the treatment of nausea and vomiting in the palliative patient: a systematic review. *J Pain Symptom Manage.* 2001;22(2):631-634.

36. dos Santos LV, Souza FH, Brunetto AT, Sasse AD, da Silveira Nogueira Lima JP. Neurokinin-1 receptor antagonists for chemotherapy-induced nausea and vomiting: a systematic review. *J Natl Cancer Inst.* 2012;104(17):1280-1292.

37. Mercadante S, Porzio G. Octreotide for malignant bowel obstruction: twenty years after. *Crit Rev Oncol Hematol.* 2012;83(3):388-392.

38. Watari H, Hosaka M, Wakui Y, et al. A prospective study on the efficacy of octreotide in the management of malignant bowel obstruction in gynecologic cancer. *Int J Gynecol Cancer*. 2012;22(4):692-696.

39. Mystakidou K, Tsilika E, Kalaidopoulou O, Chondros K, Georgaki S, Papadimitriou L. Comparison of octreotide administration vs conservative treatment in the management of inoperable bowel obstruction in patients with far advanced cancer: a randomized, double- blind, controlled clinical trial. *Anticancer Res*. 2002;22(2B):1187-1192.

40. Wood GJ, Shega JW, Lynch B, Von Roenn JH. Management of intractable nausea and vomiting in patients at the end of life: "I was feeling nauseous all of the time . . . nothing was working." *JAMA*. 2007;298(10):1196-1207.

41. von Gunten CF, Muir JC. Medical management of bowel obstruction. *Fast Facts and Concepts #45*. Milwaukee, WI: End of Life/Palliative Education Resource Center; 2008. Available at www.eperc.mcw.edu/EPERC/FastFactsIndex/ff_045.htm. Accessed December 15, 2013.

42. Kucukmetin A, Naik R, Galaal K, Bryant A, Dickinson HO. Palliative surgery versus medical management for bowel obstruction in ovarian cancer. *Cochrane Database Syst Rev*. 2010(7):CD007792.

43. Law WL, Choi HK, Chu KW. Comparison of stenting with emergency surgery as palliative treatment for obstructing primary left-sided colorectal cancer. *Br J Surg*. 2003;90(11):1429-1433.

44. Baines MJ. ABC of palliative care. Nausea, vomiting, and intestinal obstruction. *BMJ*. 1997;315(7116):1148-1150.

45. Garcia MK, McQuade J, Haddad R, et al. Systematic review of acupuncture in cancer care: a synthesis of the evidence. *J Clin Oncol*. 2013;31(7):952-960.

46. Feuer DJ, Broadley KE. Corticosteroids for the resolution of malignant bowel obstruction in advanced gynaecological and gastrointestinal cancer. *Cochrane Database Syst Rev*. 2000(2):CD001219.

47. Davis MP, Furste A. Glycopyrrolate: a useful drug in the palliation of mechanical bowel obstruction. *J Pain Symptom Manage*. 1999;18(3):153-154.

48. Sykes NP. The pathogenesis of constipation. *J Support Oncol*. 2006;4(5):213-218.

49. Goodman M, Low J, Wilkinson S. Constipation management in palliative care: a survey of practices in the United Kingdom. *J Pain Symptom Manage*. 2005;29(3):238-244.

50. Larkin PJ, Sykes NP, Centeno C, et al. The management of constipation in palliative care: clinical practice recommendations. *Palliat Med*. 2008;22(7):796-807.

51. Miles CL, Fellowes D, Goodman ML, Wilkinson S. Laxatives for the management of constipation in palliative care patients. *Cochrane Database Syst Rev*. 2006(4):CD003448.

52. Tarumi Y, Wilson MP, Szafran O, Spooner GR. Randomized, double-blind, placebo-controlled trial of oral docusate in the management of constipation in hospice patients. *J Pain Symptom Manage*. 2013;45(1):2-13.

53. Weed HG. Lactulose vs sorbitol for treatment of obstipation in hospice programs. *Mayo Clin Proc*. 2000;75(5):541.

54. Johanson JF, Morton D, Geenen J, Ueno R. Multicenter, 4-week, double-blind, randomized, placebo-controlled trial of lubiprostone, a locally-acting type-2 chloride channel activator, in patients with chronic constipation. *Am J Gastroenterol*. 2008;103(1):170-177.

55. Thomas J, Karver S, Cooney GA, et al. Methylnaltrexone for opioid-induced constipation in advanced illness. *N Engl J Med*. 2008;358(22):2332-2343.

56. Ford AC, Brenner DM, Schoenfeld PS. Efficacy of pharmacological therapies for the treatment of opioid-induced constipation: systematic review and meta-analysis. *Am J Gastroenterol*. 2013;108(10):1566-1574.

57. Gras-Miralles B, Cremonini F. A critical appraisal of lubiprostone in the treatment of chronic constipation in the elderly. *Clin Interv Aging*. 2013;8:191-200.

58. Wirz S, Nadstawek J, Elsen C, Junker U, Wartenberg HC. Laxative management in ambulatory cancer patients on opioid therapy: a prospective, open-label investigation of polyethylene glycol, sodium picosulphate and lactulose. *Eur J Cancer Care (Engl)*. 2012;21(1):131-140.

59. Lee-Robichaud H, Thomas K, Morgan J, Nelson RL. Lactulose versus polyethylene glycol for chronic constipation. *Cochrane Database Syst Rev*. 2010(7):CD007570.

FIVE

Delirium, Depression and Anxiety, Fatigue

5A | Delirium

Delirium is an acquired disturbance of attention and awareness that is accompanied by a change in baseline cognition. It develops over a short period of time—usually hours to days—and tends to fluctuate during the course of the day, often worsening at night.[1,2] Patients have reduced clarity and awareness of their environment, as well as an impaired ability to focus, sustain, or shift attention (ie, disturbance of consciousness). Cognitive changes may involve impaired memory, disorientation, and language disturbance, as well as the development of a perceptual disturbance (ie, delusions and hallucinations). Although *delirium* is the preferred term, other terms include *acute confusional state* and *encephalopathy*.

The level of psychomotor and arousal activity can vary from hyperactive (hyperalert, hypervigilant, or agitated delirium) to hypoactive (quiet or somnolent delirium), with many patients exhibiting mixed features. Motor features (eg, myoclonus, asterixis, tremors, picking at sheets) and Cheyne-Stokes respiration may be present. In palliative care, hypoactive delirium is more common (up to 80%) than hyperactive delirium and is often under-recognized because it can be mistaken for depression and fatigue.[3] The prevalence of delirium is dependent on age, underlying primary disease (eg, cancer; dementia; stroke; end-stage cardiac, pulmonary, liver, or renal disease), comorbidities (eg, baseline cognitive status, visual impairment), and the type and number of medications. The prevalence of delirium in the palliative care population ranges from 13% to 88%, depending on the underlying disease and setting and how delirium is defined.[2]

Differential Diagnosis

The differential diagnosis of delirium is broad (**Table 5.1**). Potential etiologies include general medical conditions, substance intoxications, or multiple etiologies. The most common cause of delirium in the palliative care setting is medication (eg, opioids, anticholinergics, benzodiazepines), occurring in up to 60% of patients.[4,5] The second most common cause of delirium in palliative care is metabolic insufficiency due to progressive organ failure, and the third is infection. Although other primary etiologies are sometimes uncovered (eg, hypercalcemia, deficiency states), it is more common to attribute delirium to multiple etiologies, where each factor by itself is insufficient, but collectively enough to result in delirium. Often-overlooked etiologies include constipation, urinary tract infections (UTIs), uncontrolled pain, subtle skin infections, medications, and environmental overstimulation.

Table 5.1 Differential Diagnosis of Delirium in Palliative Care

GENERAL MEDICAL CONDITION

When there is evidence from the history, physical examination, or laboratory findings that the disturbance is caused by the direct physiologic consequences of a general medical condition, consider

Metabolic	hypercalcemia, hyponatremia, renal failure, liver failure, hypothyroidism, hypoxia, hypo- or hyperglycemia
Infectious	UTI, aspiration pneumonia, cellulitis, pressure ulcers and other wounds, venous catheter infections, meningitis
Medical comorbidity	constipation or impaction, urinary retention, pulmonary embolus, myocardial infarction, stroke
Cancer-related	leptomeningeal spread, parenchymal metastasis, radiation-induced encephalopathy, paraneoplastic syndromes
Seizures	complex partial seizures, postictal states
Deficiency states	vitamin B12, thiamine, anemia
Recent surgery	invasive diagnostic procedures, minor surgeries requiring sedation, biopsies

Table 5.1 Differential Diagnosis of Delirium in Palliative Care *continued*

SUBSTANCE INTOXICATION

When there is evidence from the history, physical examination, or laboratory findings that medication use may be contributing to the delirium (as a side effect or toxic effect), consider

Medications	opioids, benzodiazepines, anticholinergic agents, antihistamines, antidepressant medications, skeletal muscle relaxants, H-2 receptor antagonists, nonsteroidal medications, corticosteroids, antiemetics with anticholinergic properties, sedative hypnotics, antiparkinson medications

MULTIPLE ETIOLOGIES

When there is evidence from the history, physical examination, or laboratory findings that the patient's delirium has more than one etiology, consider the following:

- Most often multiple etiologies exist (eg, untreated pain, constipation, UTI).
- Terminal delirium/restlessness often is a combination of progressive disease, dehydration, and accumulation of metabolites from multiorgan failure.

UTI, urinary tract infection.

Terminal delirium or *terminal restlessness* is a unique type of multifactorial delirium usually resulting from progressive disease, dehydration, and accumulation of metabolites from multiorgan failure. Terminal delirium/restlessness occurs in the final hours to weeks of life and occurs in up to 80% to 90% of patients. It is important in palliative care to distinguish between potentially reversible delirium in advanced disease and terminal delirium/restlessness, which is part of the dying process but may still require symptomatic treatment for patient comfort.

Prognosis

Older patients with an episode of delirium have a 1-year mortality of up to 50%, and the risk will increase the longer the delirium episode persists.[6] However, the prognostic implications of a delirium depend on the underlying primary disease, the etiology of the delirium, and the stage of illness. At one extreme, neurocognitive symptoms (as part of a terminal delirium/restlessness), along with declines in performance status and nutritional limitations, are known to be predictive of approaching death. At the other extreme, delirium is a completely reversible process that is independent of survival (eg, opioid-induced delirium in early-stage cancer). In reality, the prognostic importance of delirium in advanced disease lies somewhere between these two extremes and may present as a dip in the functional trajectory curve with less than full recovery to a patient's baseline. Therefore, delirium is often not reversible and estimates of reversibility (variably defined) range from 20% to 50%.[4] Even when delirium is reversible, the course of recovery may take days to weeks depending on the severity of the delirium and underlying cognitive deficits. Delirium due to medications and nonrespiratory infections are more likely reversible than those due to progressive underlying organ failure.

Management

History and Examination

The cornerstone of a change-in-mental-status consult is a complete history and examination (including rectal examination) with detailed medication review. A high index of suspicion is needed, particularly because the hypoactive variant can be unrecognized and undiagnosed. It is important to obtain collateral history from family and other providers, as well as to review all medications and dosages in the several days preceding the onset of symptoms. Comparing home medications with current medications may reveal a discrepancy contributing to altered mental status. Simple tests of attention (eg, spell "world" backwards, count from 100 by 7s) often are useful in making the diagnosis, though patients with advanced illness may not be able to participate in formal mental status exams. A variety of screening scales can potentially assist in the diagnosis of delirium (eg, Delirium Rating Scale, Confusion Assessment Method [or CAM-ICU], Memorial Delirium-Assessment Scale),[7] but they do not substitute for a thorough and well-conducted history and physical examination. Vital signs (eg, fever, blood pressure, oxygen saturation), motor signs (eg, myoclonus, asterixis), and focal neurological deficits also assist in the diagnosis.

Diagnostic Work-Up

The diagnostic work-up will depend on the goals of care, which, in turn, will depend on the patient's wishes and prognosis and the benefits and burdens of each test, coupled with the condition's potential reversibility. Low-burden investigations in the hospital setting may include vital signs; oxygen saturation; routine X rays; electroencephalograms; urinalysis and urine culture; and blood draws for chemistries (including liver function and blood glucose), hematology, toxicology, and cultures. Higher-burden investigations include lumbar punctures, MRIs, and other invasive diagnostic procedures. The unexpected onset of delirium in patients with only moderately advanced disease should nearly always trigger a screen for potentially reversible causes of incipient dementia (eg, vitamin B12 and thyroid function studies). In solid tumor patients, tests for ionized calcium to rule out hypercalcemia and brain imaging to rule out metastasis should be considered, except in terminal stages of disease.

To accurately establish the diagnosis of delirium and to distinguish it from dementia, depression, psychosis, mania, anxiety, and aphasia, one should consider consulting a specialist (eg, neurology, psychiatry, geriatrics). After the diagnosis of delirium is established, it should be further categorized as hyperactive, hypoactive, or mixed. Particularly in palliative care, hypoactive delirium can be mistaken for depression. **Finally, and most importantly, one should step back and place the delirium in the context of the overall disease process** (ie, delirium in advanced disease, terminal delirium) and estimate the survival prognosis in days to weeks, weeks to months, or longer. There are many similarities between the spectrum of unsettled behaviors in terminal delirium/restlessness and delirium in advanced disease. Therefore, make sure a diagnosis of terminal delirium is not premature or caused by medication used for symptom control (eg, narcotics, anxiolytics, antisecretory agents). Likewise, an extensive work-up for reversible causes in the final hours of life should be carefully avoided.

Educate Family and Staff

Delirium can be highly distressing to family members, and considerable effort is required to educate them about etiology, prognosis, and management. Families and loved ones often experience a *double bereavement*; first the loss of a meaningful connection when the patient is delirious, and then the loss of a loved one when death occurs. Education should include informing the family that fluctuations in mental status are to be expected and that symptoms often are worse at night. Acknowledging and validating the ups and downs that delirium introduces can help (eg, "This is a roller-coaster ride and there will be good days and bad days."), as well as emphasizing that most patients have limited or no recollection of their symptoms after the episode subsides. Part of the discussion should include estimates of prognosis, a summary of uncertainties that exist, and continuous re-evaluation of the patient's clinical situation over time. Family, caregivers, and provider staff often need additional support to reinforce the goals of care and to anticipate the possibility of gradual deterioration to an active dying phase.

Etiology-Specific Delirium Treatment

Table 5.2 lists causes of delirium that might respond favorably to specific treatments. **The most important potential reversible etiologies include medication-induced delirium, infections, hypercalcemia, constipation, and undertreated pain.** Many of the etiologies, although potentially treatable, signify advancing disease. Careful review of medications and avoiding polypharmacy cannot be overemphasized. Dehydration can be relieved by oral (PO), intravenous (IV), or subcutaneous (SC) hydration (hypodermoclysis), but the utility of rehydration improving mental status and energy levels in the final days of life has been disappointing.[8] These treatments should be tailored to the individual's needs and the goals of the patient and family. Many potential treatments should involve time-limited trials with specific time periods, targets, and plans to reevaluate.

Table 5.2 Etiology-Specific Management of Delirium

ETIOLOGY	TREATMENT	COMMENT
Opioid toxicity	Reduce dosage, if practical, or change to another opioid (opioid rotation)	A common cause of delirium in the palliative care setting; motor signs may be present (eg, myoclonus)
Other drugs	Stop, wean, or decrease possible offending drug (eg, anticholinergic agents, antisecretory agents, anxiolytics, steroids, antiepileptic drugs)	High index of suspicion needed; withdrawing some drugs abruptly can also cause delirium (eg, benzodiazepines, stimulants, barbiturates)
Progressive organ failure: renal, liver, cardiac, dementia	Treatments often limited or involve considerable trade-offs (eg, dialysis, transplantation)	Second most common cause of delirium in palliative care setting; less likely to be reversible over the long term
Infections: UTI, aspiration pneumonia, sepsis, decubitus ulcers	Work-up and antibiotics depending on the goals of care; short course of oral antibiotics may be adequate	Third most common cause of delirium in palliative care setting; UTIs often overlooked as a cause
Hypoxia	Treat underlying cause and administer oxygen	Oxygen is commonly applied in hospitals whether beneficial or not; high concentrations may require expensive set ups at home (eg, liquid O_2 delivery apparatus)
Deficiency states	Multivitamins, B vitamins, hypothyroidism	Uncommon except in cases of advanced alcoholism and severe malnutrition
Constipation/urinary retention	Rectal examination, abdominal X ray, disimpaction, laxatives, catheterization	Often overlooked as a cause; prevention much less burdensome than treatment
Hypercalcemia	Intravenous hydration and bisphosphonates	Although potentially reversible, treatments are expensive and burdensome at home; often signifies advancing disease
Complex partial seizures	Antiepileptic medication	Often signifies advancing disease
Pain	Adjust/rotate pain medications	See chapter 2.
Brain metastases/primary brain tumor progression	Steroids, radiotherapy, surgery	Treatment may aggravate symptoms and be of high burden for the potential benefit

UTI, urinary tract infection.

Supportive Care and Managing Behaviors

Agitation and combative behavior are some of the most challenging aspects of delirium treatment. Interpersonal or environmental manipulations may be useful for mild to moderate agitation. These include quiet reassurance in soft voices, frequent orienting cues (eg, clocks, lights on and off at proper times), family member presence, optimizing sensory input (eg, hearing aids, glasses), and minimizing ambient noise levels and night disruption. Although particularly important for geriatric patients, these interventions have a role for all patients. Physical restraints should be used only very rarely and, if used, should be time limited and accompanied with clear documentation in the medical record that other methods have been tried and have failed.

Pharmacologic Treatment of Symptoms

When strategies to prevent or reverse delirium are unsuccessful or inappropriate, pharmacotherapy can help calm the patient and improve mentation (**Table 5.3**).[3,9-12] Antipsychotic agents are the treatment of choice. Although comparative data are sparse, haloperidol is generally preferred as a first-line medication because it has few anticholinergic side effects, is available in oral and parenteral formulations, has fewer active metabolites, and has a relatively small risk of hypotension and extrapyramidal side effects (over the short term). High dosages may be required. Existing data indicate no superiority of second-generation antipsychotics (ie, risperidone, olanzapine, quetiapine) over haloperidol for managing delirium. They are generally safe and may have fewer extrapyramidal side effects compared with haloperidol, however these medications generally are more expensive than haloperidol. There are limited data for the use of ziprasidone and aripiprazole for this indication. All of the conventional and atypical antipsychotic agents carry a black box warning of increased mortality in dementia-related psychosis (see note at base of Table 5.3).

Benzodiazepines should be used cautiously (if at all) for delirium and are usually reserved for withdrawal from alcohol or sedative hypnotics, although they may be useful in severe agitation or for those who cannot tolerate antipsychotic agents or are at high risk for seizures. For

Table 5.3 Pharmacologic Treatment for Delirium in Palliative Care

MEDICATION	DOSAGE	COMMENT
Antipsychotic Medications*		
Haloperidol*	1 mg PO or 0.5 mg IV/SC (parenteral dosages are twice as potent as oral dosages) and can be given hourly as needed, then every 6 to 12 hours in divided doses; titrate to higher dosages for patients who continue to be agitated	Preferred medication; may need 5 mg SC every 6 hours for severe symptoms. Generally, parenteral doses are twice as potent as oral doses.
Chlorpromazine*	25 mg-50 mg PO/IV hourly until calm, then every 6 to 12 hours or by infusion	Consider if more sedation is needed; can cause hypotension
Risperidone*	0.25 mg-0.5 mg PO every 12 hours, titrated to 1.5 mg every 12 hours	More expensive; dosages up to 4 mg-6 mg daily have been used
Olanzapine*	2.5 mg-5 mg PO daily, titrated to 5 mg-10 mg daily	More expensive; dosages up to 15 mg-20 mg daily have been used
Quetiapine*	12.5 mg-25 mg PO every 12 hours, titrated to 100 mg every 12 hours	More expensive; dosages up to 300 mg-400 mg daily have been used
Benzodiazepines		
Lorazepam	0.5 mg-1 mg PO/SL/IV/SC/PR hourly until calm	Reserved for more severe cases or when seizures or alcohol withdrawal are suspected.
Psychostimulants		
Methylphenidate	2.5 mg-5 mg every morning and at noon; adjust gradually upward as needed if beneficial, to a maximum of 60 mg per day	Has been used for patients with hypoactive delirium; limited evidence regarding efficacy. Use with caution in those with a history of anxiety, tachycardia, or arrythmia.

*US Food and Drug Administration black box warning for antipsychotic medications: Not approved for dementia-related psychosis. Elderly patients with dementia-related psychosis treated with either typical or atypical antipsychotic drugs are at an increased risk of death and possibly stroke compared with placebo patients. Most deaths are due to either cardiovascular or infectious events. There is also a potential for metabolic adverse effects with prolonged use.

Depending on the goals of care, patients receiving antipsychotic medications for delirium may benefit from electrocardiographic monitoring, given the potential for QTc prolongation and Torsade de pointes. In this situation, the risks versus benefits of the medications need to be discussed with the family, as these potential adverse effects may or may not be outweighed by the need for symptom control at the end of life.

some patients, benzodiazepines can cause a paradoxical agitation and worsen the symptoms of delirium. Methylphenidate has shown favorable effects in hypoactive delirium, although evidence is limited. Cholinesterase inhibitors have been shown to be ineffective in delirium.

Finally, a small minority of patients with agitated terminal delirium will have persistent and troubling symptoms despite the use of antipsychotic agents and conventional dosages of benzodiazepines. In such circumstances, increasing doses of sedatives can be used, with the possibility of needing proportionate palliative sedation, possibly to unconsciousness (see chapters 8 and 9). Providers must be very clear that the intention is to relieve symptoms and not to hasten death. The family or decision maker should agree with the plan. All parties involved must understand the details and justification for use of sedating medications to respond to terminal delirium.

5B | Depression and Anxiety

Periodic feelings of depression and anxiety are normal and expected consequences of the uncertainties of severe illness and approaching death; however, high levels of persistent anxiety or depression are not an inevitable part of serious illness or the dying process.[13-16] It is important to avoid overnormalizing (eg, "Of course he is anxious and depressed — he is dying!") or overpathologizing (eg, "She is crying, so we better put her on medication for depression."). The need to medically treat depression and anxiety depends on their intensity, persistence, and disruption of basic life functioning. Treatment should be considered when these effects dominate other emotions and interfere with the ability to enjoy other aspects of life. Clinical syndromes of anxiety or depression may be amenable to intervention even when the underlying disease no longer can be treated. In this circumstance, treatment of depression or anxiety may be one of the most important interventions to enhance a patient's quality of life.[17]

Assessment

Depression

Depression can be effectively treated if it is recognized. Two simple questions have been found to have good sensitivity to screen for depression. A more formal exploration is indicated if the patient gives a positive answer to either of these questions[18,19]:

- Are you depressed? (Screening for patient awareness of depression)
- Do you have much interest or pleasure in doing things? (Screening for anhedonia)

Normal sadness and grief are directly connected to and proportionate with the patient's loss, and the capacity for pleasure in some aspects of life is retained. Clinical depression is more generalized and unremitting and may be associated with hopelessness, helplessness, worthlessness, and guilt.[15] Patients may also experience disproportionate dysphoria, tearfulness, anger, or social withdrawal. Both groups of patients may think about death, but clinically depressed patients may become preoccupied with death and begin to plan for it in ways inconsistent with past values. Terminally ill patients with depression are at higher risk of suicide and suicidal ideation, and they may have increased desires and requests for hastened death (see chapter 8). Because many of the symptoms of severe illness may overlap with symptoms of depression (ie, fatigue, anorexia, sleep disturbance, poor concentration, social withdrawal, hopelessness),[19] consultation from an experienced psychiatrist or psychologist may be helpful in uncertain or complex cases (**Table 5.4**). Because clinical depression is prevalent in the terminally ill and is amenable to treatment, clinicians should have a high index of suspicion.

Anxiety

A careful history and physical examination are the most important first steps for providing effective interventions to treat anxiety. Initial emphasis should be placed on identifying treatable medical complications (eg, pain, dyspnea, fear, anxiety caused by medications), but a high level of suspicion should be maintained for other frequently occurring contributing factors such as physical, psychological, social, and spiritual pain.

Table 5.4 Causes and Symptoms of Depression

CAUSES

Psychiatric

- Major depression
- Adjustment disorders
- Association with anxiety disorders, particularly panic disorder

Medical

- Poorly controlled pain or other physical symptoms (eg, dyspnea, nausea, insomnia)
- Drugs (eg, opioids, corticosteroids, diazepam, interferon)
- Tumor involvement of central nervous system
- Pancreatic cancer
- Metabolic disturbances (eg, abnormal levels of sodium or calcium)
- Nutritional problems (eg, anemia or deficiencies in vitamin B12 or folate)
- Endocrine disorders (eg, hypothyroidism or adrenal insufficiency)
- Neurological disorders (eg, Parkinson's disease)
- Infections (eg, urinary tract infections)

Psychological, social, and spiritual

- Grief
- Existential distress
- Concerns about family
- Overwhelming financial or family distress
- Hopelessness and meaninglessness
- Guilt about past wrongdoing
- Fear of expressing anger

LOOK FOR

Psychological indicators

- Profound feelings or thoughts of worthlessness
- Excessive feelings of guilt
- Anhedonia
- Wishing for death
- Hopelessness and helplessness
- Suicidal ideation
- Personal history of depression or substance abuse

Somatic signs and symptoms

- Less valuable when assessing depression in terminally ill patients; the illness itself can produce symptoms of fatigue, loss of energy, anorexia, and insomnia

Anxiety symptoms (**Table 5.5**) may be triggered by a range of medical transitions, such as the initial diagnosis of serious illness, a recurrence, treatment side effects or failure, or discussion of hospice. The patient may have a range of stated or unstated fears that also may trigger symptoms of anxiety (eg, uncontrolled pain, isolation, abandonment, loss of control, worrying about a spouse or child, being a burden, death, dying).

Anxiety disorders are common in the general population, and these underlying conditions are likely to be aggravated in transition periods when a patient has a serious, potentially fatal medical condition. Fortunately, anxiety disorders are very treatable once recognized. The most common anxiety disorders are listed here:

- **Adjustment disorder with anxious mood:** The anxiety will be directly related to and triggered by the stressful event (in this case, directly related to the serious, potentially terminal illness).
- **Generalized anxiety disorder[20]:** The anxiety is continuously present and will have preceded the diagnosis of the new serious illness; the dominant symptoms are continuous tenseness, worry, and irritability.
- **Panic disorder:** Panic disorder is characterized by episodic panic attacks (unexpected and unprovoked attacks of severe cognitive and physical symptoms of anxiety) with a high state of vigilance in between (anticipatory anxiety); if unrecognized or undertreated, it may be associated with phobic behavior.
- **Mixed anxiety and depression:** Anxiety and depression frequently coexist with overlapping symptoms (eg, sleep disturbance, difficulty concentrating, irritability, and fatigue); treatment should be targeted to the dominant symptoms.

Treatment

The treatment of both anxiety and depression depends on a careful assessment and treatment of underlying cause(s) and frequently involves a combination of supportive/existential psychotherapy, structured cognitive therapy, and pharmacological treatments. Members of the multidisciplinary team may be involved, depending on the nature of the symptoms and the patient's underlying disease and prognosis. Several factors need to be considered when designing a treatment plan:

Table 5.5 Causes and Symptoms of Anxiety

CAUSES

Situational

Worry about family, finances

Fear of the unknown, hospital, treatment

Isolation, inadequate support

Role loss, sense of uselessness

Uncertainty, lack of information, misinformation

Caused by drugs

Corticosteroids

Drug-induced hallucinations

Benzodiazepines or opioids

Psychostimulants

Albuterol

Withdrawal states precipitated by abrupt discontinuation of benzodiazepines, alcohol, opioids

Organic

Uncontrolled pain and other symptoms

Dyspnea, hypoxia, increasing respiratory effort

Weakness

Hypoglycemia, hyperthyroidism sepsis, fever, hypertension

Insomnia

Brain tumor

Adverse drug reactions such as akathisia or myoclonus

Psychological

Denial, anger, guilt, fear

Preexisting anxiety disorders (eg, exagger-ated reaction)

LOOK FOR

Persistent tenseness

Inability to relax

Worry, fearfulness, dread

More than normal mood variation

Poor concentration

Impaired ability to assimilate or recall information

Rumination, intrusive thoughts

Indecisiveness

Insomnia

Irritability, restlessness

Inability to distract self and be distracted

Panic attacks

Sweating, tremor

- the patient's subjective level of distress, symptom severity, and functional impairment
- duration of the distress
- the family's reaction to the patient's distress and their coping resources
- presence of uncontrolled symptoms, particularly pain (ie, physical, psychosocial, or spiritual)
- benefits versus burdens of potential treatments
- the strengths and resources of the multidisciplinary team
- the patient's and family's preferences and past experiences.

Short-Term Counseling for Anxiety and Depression

If short-term counseling is initiated to help relieve anxiety and depression, family members should be included when appropriate, and emphasis should be placed on the following:

- providing as much updated information about treatment and prognosis as the patient desires
- correcting misconceptions about the past and present with honest and compassionate communication
- educating patients and family members about the psychological, biological, and pharmacological factors that contribute to anxiety and depression
- securing supportive relationships and helping the patient reestablish a renewed sense of self-worth and meaning during the terminal stage of illness
- establishing attainable short-term goals and expectations
- identifying and emphasizing a patient's past strengths and successful coping techniques, including distraction, short-term psychotherapy, journaling, and exercise
- teaching relaxation techniques, such as focusing on passive breathing (the natural rhythms of breathing), accompanied by either passive or active muscle relaxation, meditation, guided imagery, or self-hypnosis to help reduce anxiety and increase the patient's sense of control—massage and music therapy[21] have a special role in treating anxiety disorders in the palliative care population

- providing ongoing emotional support and caring presence to reduce the patient's sense of isolation
- judiciously using lighthearted humor.

The treatment of these disorders in the severely medically ill is believed to be similar to its treatment in other clinical settings,[16,22,23] with a few caveats:

- interpersonal psychotherapy must be adapted to the patient's energy level, cognitive status, and prognosis
- side effects may preclude use of some or all traditional pharmacological agents (**Table 5.6** and **Table 5.7**)
- starting doses may need to be adjusted downward depending on illness severity
- selective serotonin reuptake inhibitors (SSRIs) are less sedating and more stimulating, but they may increase nausea, aggravate anxiety, cause sexual dysfunction, and increase insomnia in the short term
- tricyclic antidepressants (TCAs) are especially useful if neuropathic pain or insomnia are part of the picture, but the need for gradual dose titration and anticholinergic side effects may limit their use
- TCAs and SSRIs may take up to 4 or more weeks to work for depression and anxiety.

TCAs and SSRIs both carry an FDA black box warning for increased risk of suicide in children, adolescents, and young adults with major depressive or other psychiatric disorders. In patients older than 65 years, depression and certain other psychiatric disorders are associated with increased suicidal risk. Observe all patients for clinical worsening, suicidality, or unusual behavioral changes. Advise families and caregivers of the need for close observation and communication with prescriber.

Psychostimulants have a special role for terminally ill patients with depression and fatigue because of their rapid onset and their immediately energizing effects.[24,25] For patients with life expectancy less than 4 to 6 weeks, psychostimulants may be preferable given their more rapid onset of action.

Benzodiazepines are useful in the acute treatment of patients with severe anxiety because of their rapid onset of action and ability to provide immediate relief; benzodiazepines also can be overused when counseling would be more appropriate or when more direct treatment of pain, dyspnea, or depression would be more effective.

Consider a psychiatric referral in the following situations: uncertainty about the diagnosis, patient unresponsiveness to first-line therapy, preexisting psychiatric disease or current symptoms of psychosis, patient inability to swallow previously effective psychiatric medications, or patient who is suicidal or persistently requesting a hastened death (see sections 8C [p. 180] and 8D [p. 184]).

Table 5.6 Selected Pharmacological Agents for Treating Major Depression in Patients with Advanced Disease

DRUG	DOSAGE STARTING DOSE (S) DOSAGE RANGE (R)	NOTES
Selective serotonin reuptake inhibitors (SSRIs): Sedation and dry mouth are less common than with tricyclic agents; less likely to alleviate neuropathic pain; often reduce libido		
Escitalopram	S: 5 mg every morning or every evening R: 5 mg-20 mg	Fewer drug-drug interactions Potential for QT prolongation
Citalopram	S: 10 mg every morning or every evening R: 10 mg-40 mg	Fewer drug-drug interactions Potential for QT prolongation; maximum dosage in patients >60 years is 20 mg daily
Fluoxetine	S: 5 mg-10 mg every morning R: 5 mg-80 mg	Avoid in patients with hepatic impairment due to long half-life Taper off when discontinuing Significant drug-drug interactions
Paroxetine	S: 10 mg every evening R: 10 mg-40 mg	More sedating Significant drug-drug interactions Due to short half-life, most concerning for withdrawal among SSRIs

continued

Table 5.6 Selected Pharmacological Agents for Treating Major Depression in Patients with Advanced Disease *continued*

DRUG	DOSAGE STARTING DOSE (S) DOSAGE RANGE (R)	NOTES
Sertraline	S: 12.5 mg-25 mg every morning R: 25 mg-200 mg	For frail elderly, begin with half the usual starting dose
Tricyclic antidepressants: *Give in a single dose, usually at bedtime; helpful for insomnia and neuropathic pain; anticholinergic side effects. Often not as well tolerated as SSRIs*		
Nortriptyline	S: 10 mg at bedtime R: 10 mg-150 mg	Oral solution available; can monitor drug levels Fewer anticholinergic side effects than amitriptyline and therefore more likely to be tolerated in elderly patients
Amitriptyline	S: 10 mg-25 mg at bedtime R: 10 mg-150 mg	Sedating; anticholinergic side effects often limiting
Selective serotonin/norepinephrine reuptake inhibitors (SNRIs): *May increase energy and act as adjuncts for neuropathic pain; often reduce libido*		
Venlafaxine	S: 18.75 mg-37.5 mg every morning or twice daily R: 75 mg-150 mg twice daily	Available in extended-release formulation starting at 37.5 mg every morning or twice daily, with range of 75 mg-100 mg twice daily Taper off when discontinuing; withdrawal can occur with even a few missed doses
Duloxetine	S: 10 mg-20 mg every morning or twice daily R: 20 mg-60 mg every morning or twice daily	May be useful for coexistent generalized anxiety; neuromodulator effects may be useful for treatment of coexisting neuropathic pain
Miscellaneous antidepressants: *Can be very useful for some patients with anxiety or low energy levels; cost may be a consideration*		
Mirtazapine	S: 7.5 mg-15 mg at bedtime R: 15 mg-60 mg	Norepinephrine and serotonin antagonist; possible sedation (may be beneficial in those with trouble falling asleep), weight gain (a potential benefit), agranulocytosis (0.1%)

Table 5.6 Selected Pharmacological Agents for Treating Major Depression in Patients with Advanced Disease *continued*

DRUG	DOSAGE	NOTES
	STARTING DOSE (S) DOSAGE RANGE (R)	
Trazodone	S: 12.5 mg-25 mg at bedtime R: 50 mg-300 mg	Sedating properties may be helpful for insomnia
Psychostimulants: *Rapid effect but may exacerbate anxiety and restlessness; taper off slowly if possible*		
Methylphenidate	S: 2.5 mg-5 mg at 8 am and noon R: 10 mg-60 mg in divided doses	Doses greater than 30 mg per day are not usually necessary, but occasionally patients require up to 60 mg per day; transdermal patches, oral liquids, and chewable tablets are available. Side effects including nervousness and agitation may be dose-limiting. Avoid use in cardiac patients with preexisting arrythmia and those with seizure history.
Modafinil	S: 100 mg every morning R: 100 mg-200 mg	May have less abuse potential than amphetamines
Benzodiazepines: *Helpful when anxiety coexists with depression (Table 5.7)*		

Table 5.7 Medications Used to Treat Acute Anxiety in Patients with Advanced Disease

DRUG	DOSAGE	NOTES
Benzodiazepines: *Effective in providing immediate relief for acute anxiety symptoms; side effects include sedation, cognitive slowing, and physical dependence, limiting use of these drugs for patients already in low energy or confused states*		
Short half-life		
Alprazolam	0.25 mg-2 mg PO or SL three or four times per day	Peak 30 minutes; liquid available; other routes: SL/PR; duration 4 to 6 hours; half-life 6 to 27 hours; high potential for rebound anxiety in between doses; uneven effect with chronic use because of short half-life

continued

Table 5.7 Medications Used to Treat Acute Anxiety in Patients with Advanced Disease *continued*

DRUG	DOSAGE	NOTES
Medium half-life		
Lorazepam	0.5 mg-1.5 mg PO two to four times per day	Peak 5 to 20 minutes; liquid available; other routes: SL/PR/IV; duration 6 to 8 hours; half-life 13 to 15 hours
Long half-life		
Clonazepam	0.25 mg-2 mg PO two or three times per day	Peak 20 to 60 minutes; other routes: SL/PR/dissolvable wafer; duration 12 hours; half-life 19 to 50 hours
Diazepam	2 mg-10 mg PO two to four times per day	Peak 15 to 45 minutes; liquid available; other routes: SL/PR/IV; half-life 20 to 50 hours, but active metabolites half-life 50 to 100 hours; high potential for accumulation and oversedation

Nonbenzodiazepine anxiolytic: Generally less effective for anxiety disorders than benzodiazepines, but may have some use for patients intolerant to benzodiazepines or with past addiction problems; common side effects include dizziness, headache, drowsiness, light-headedness, fatigue, nausea, insomnia, and restlessness; will not prevent benzodiazepine withdrawal

Buspirone	5 mg-10 mg two or three times per day	Peak 0.7 to 1.5 hours; tablets only; half-life 2 to 11 hours; delayed onset and use in chronic anxiety states limits its use in the palliative care setting

Major tranquilizers: Severe acute anxiety associated with paranoia, severe agitation, hallucinations, delirium, or confused states

Haloperidol	0.5 mg-5 mg every 2 to 12 hours	Peak 2 to 6 hours; liquid available; other routes: SL/PR/SC/IV (parenteral dosage twice as potent as oral dosage); neuroleptic; antiemetic benefit
		Carries FDA black box warning for use in dementia-related psychosis, see Table 5.3.

Selective serotonin reuptake inhibitors and tricyclic antidepressants also are used to treat chronic anxiety disorders and mixed anxiety-depression in doses similar to those used for depression. See Table 5.6 for usual starting doses and dose ranges.

IV, intranevous; PO, oral; PR, rectal; SC, subcutaneous; SL, sublingual.

5C | Fatigue

Fatigue is one of the most common symptoms encountered by providers in the palliative care population. Prevalence estimates of fatigue range from 48% to as high as 80%.[26,27] Reported prevalence rates are highest among those with cancer, although those with chronic heart or lung disease, HIV, and neurologic diseases such as multiple sclerosis and stroke may also suffer from significant fatigue. *Fatigue* has been defined as a "subjective feeling of tiredness, weakness, or lack of energy"[26] and may have both physical and cognitive dimensions; it also may be among the most severe of symptoms reported by patients. Physical fatigue (weakness) may prevent patients from participating in everyday activities such as cooking and exercising; cognitive fatigue (tiredness) may prevent patients from enjoying activities such as reading or driving a car.

Fatigue can either be primary or secondary.[28] Primary fatigue is directly related to the disease mechanism, whereas secondary fatigue is related to non–disease-specific factors. There are many diseases in palliative care in which primary fatigue is likely to occur, including cancer, HIV/AIDS, stroke, heart failure, rheumatoid arthritis, systemic lupus erthymatosis, and Parkinson's disease. The pathophysiology of primary fatigue is not well understood, although many factors are possible in a given disease. These include centrally mediated processes (eg, attentional deficit resulting from damage to the reticular formation and related structures involved in the subcortical attentional network), immunological factors (eg, effect of proinflammatory cytokines), neuroendocrine involvement (eg, hypothalamic-pituitary-adrenal dysregulation), and peripheral abnormalities (eg, alterations in muscle metabolism).

When evaluating a patient with fatigue, the first step is to perform a comprehensive history and physical examination with a detailed review of medications and treatments to establish that the fatigue is not caused by a potentially reversible condition (secondary fatigue). If fatigue persists after contributing causes have been ruled out and treated, symptomatic treatments should be considered.

History and Examination

Key aspects of the history when evaluating a patient with fatigue include an assessment of the intensity and duration of fatigue as well as the impact of fatigue on activities of everyday life. Subjective fatigue (or tiredness) can be measured and followed over time on a 10-point rating scale as part of general assessment tools such as the Edmonton Symptom Assessment Scale Revised (ESAS-R; www.palliative.org/newpc/_pdfs/tools/ESAS-r%20guidelines.pdf). In addition, several validated instruments for the measurement of fatigue are available.[28] The Fatigue Severity Scale (FSS) measures the impact of fatigue on functioning and is not specific to any particular disease; it is brief and reports a single score rather than a detailed qualitative assessment. The Multidimensional Fatigue Inventory (MFI-20) is comprehensive and reports on many dimensions of fatigue, such as general fatigue, mental fatigue, motivation, and activity. These scales may be useful for following fatigue scores over time, but subjective patient assessment should continue to be used whenever possible. It is also important to screen for depression and anxiety and to inquire about sleep quality; patients may complain of a persistent sense of tiredness that is not relieved by rest. Providers should also ask patients whether any changes in medications have been made recently, particularly in regard to increases in opioid dosages.

Physical examination should be comprehensive and should include measurement of orthostatic blood pressure, assessment of mucous membranes for pallor or icterus, and an evaluation for lymphadenopathy, murmurs, or bruits. A detailed neurological examination, including testing for cognition, should be performed.

Secondary Fatigue

Always search for contributing causes before concluding that fatigue is a manifestation of the disease itself (**Table 5.8**). Treatment of these causes should be individualized and consistent with patient goals of care. Anemia is a common cause of fatigue in cancer patients (both treatment-related and as a result of the disease process) and in patients with other chronic diseases such as congestive heart failure and chronic

Table 5.8 Secondary Fatigue: Causes, Evaluation, and Treatment*

CAUSE	EVALUATION	TREATMENT
Anemia	Complete blood count, iron studies, vitamin B12	Erythropoetic agents Transfusion Iron/B12 supplementation
Infection/fever	Urine/blood cultures, chest X ray, if appropriate	Antibiotics/antipyretics
Cachexia/anorexia	Albumin, prealbumin	Little evidence for nutritional supplements or megestrol acetate
Dehydration/electrolyte imbalance	Orthostatic blood pressure, electrolyte panel	Hydration, electrolyte supplementation; bisphosphonates, if indicated
Hypothyroidism	Thyroid studies	Thyroid hormone supplementation as indicated
Mood disorders/depression	Refer to discussion on pp. 100-110.	Antidepressant medications as appropriate
Sleep disturbance	Sleep hygiene assessment	Consider sedative agents at bedtime
Opioid-induced neurotoxicty	Evaluate recent medication changes, dosage adjustments	Consider reducing opioid dosage or rotating to a different opioid, or symptomatic treatment (discussed below)
Untreated pain	Detailed pain assessment	Adjustment of pain medications (see chapter 2); consider opioid rotation or addition of adjuvant medication
Other medications/polypharmacy	Comprehensive review of medications	Discontinue or reduce dosages of medications (such as anticholinergics or benzodiazepines) that may be contributing to fatigue
Adverse effects of treatment	Radiation/chemotherapy	Consider whether disease-directed treatments (such as chemotherapy for cancer or interferon for multiple sclerosis) are leading to worsening symptoms, and reduce or discontinue based on goals of care

*Treatment should be individualized and use of more invasive treatments such as intravenous hydration, intravenous antibiotics, and nutrition should be consistent with goals of care.

kidney disease (CKD). Epoetin alfa and darbepoetin alfa may help with anemia, but both now carry FDA black box warnings for increased mortality and tumor progression in cancer patients and increased mortality and serious cardiovascular events in CKD patients. Red cell transfusions have been used for symptomatic treatment of fatigue related to anemia, but treatment should be individualized; transfusions are costly and not without risk, and the effects may be of short duration. Antibiotics and antipyretics may be used for treatment of fatigue related to infection or fever, if consistent with the patient's goals of care. Cachexia may be associated with a sensation of fatigue, but there is little evidence that increasing caloric intake or nutritional supplementation with polyunsaturated fatty acid or eicosapentanoic acid are of benefit. Megestrol acetate has been shown to improve appetite in cancer patients when compared with placebo but has not been shown to significantly improve fatigue.[26] This medication increases the risk for thrombosis and is not indicated for patients at risk for clotting. Hypogonadism in cancer patients has been associated with low mood and fatigue,[29] but short trials of IM testosterone for quality-of-life improvement in this population have been disappointing.[30] Screening for depression is discussed earlier in this chapter and treatment with antidepressants may lead to a subjective improvement of fatigue. Opioid-induced neurotoxicity also should be considered as a cause of fatigue, and opioid rotation or dose reduction may be recommended in these patients. Untreated pain also should not be overlooked as a cause of fatigue and should be treated appropriately.

Pharmacological Treatment of Fatigue

If a specific source or cause of fatigue is not identified, symptomatic treatments for fatigue should be considered on an individualized basis.[31] Most of the research to date has concentrated on stimulant medications such as methylphenidate (which carries an FDA black box warning for drug dependence), although short-term treatment with a corticosteroid such as dexamethasone may be helpful, if tolerated (**Table 5.9**). Modafinil acts via inhibition of gamma-aminobutyric acid, thus promoting release of excitatory neurotransmitters, and recent research suggests that it is an effective treatment for fatigue.[32] Donepezil is a centrally acting cholinesterase inhibitor currently approved for symptomatic treatment of Alzheimer's disease, although there is some evidence that it may be useful for treatment of opioid-induced fatigue.[33]

Amantadine has been suggested as a treatment for fatigue in multiple sclerosis patients, but it may be poorly tolerated, and there is little evidence that it is effective at reducing fatigue levels.[34] Open-label studies of L-carnitine supplementation in cancer patients with L-carnitine deficiency have demonstrated an improvement in fatigue, although the research in this area is still being conducted and no established guidelines or doses are available.[35] L-carnitine also may be effective for the treatment of fatigue in patients with multiple sclerosis.[36]

Table 5.9 Pharmacological Treatment of Fatigue

MEDICATION	DOSAGE	COMMENTS
Methylphenidate	Start at 2.5 mg-5 mg at 8 am and noon, titrate to 10 mg-60 mg daily in divided doses	Side effects including nervousness and agitation may be dose-limiting; avoid use in cardiac patients with preexisting arrhythmia
		FDA black box warning for drug dependence
Modafinil	Start at 100 mg every morning and consider titration to 200 mg every morning, except in those with liver failure	May reduce opioid-induced sedation[26] and reduce fatigue in those with cancer[32]
Corticosteroids	Start dexamethasone 8 mg per day in divided doses (give last dose midday to prevent insomnia)	Some data on effectiveness[37]; may be useful for short-term treatment of fatigue
Donepezil	Start at 5 mg every morning	May be useful for opioid-induced sedation
Amantadine	Start at 100 mg twice a day[36]	May be useful for fatigue in those with multiple sclerosis, although use may be limited by GI or CNS side effects

CNS, central nervous system; FDA, US Food and Drug Administration; GI, gastrointestinal.

Nonpharmacological Treatment of Fatigue

Nonpharmacological interventions for fatigue such as massage, music therapy, aromatherapy, and psychotherapy/relaxation therapy should also be considered and tried if available. Educating patients on proper sleep hygiene may help to improve sleep quality and reduce daytime fatigue. Physical and occupational therapy evaluations also should be considered to help patients cope and adjust to the impact of fatigue on their enjoyment of physical activities. Focused psychosocial interventions that are designed to educate patients about fatigue and teach them coping mechanisms also have been shown to be helpful.[38]

Further Discussion

Delirium

1. What are the key differences between delirium and dementia?
2. What are the key differences between agitated delirium (hyperactive) and quiet delirium (hypoactive)? Which is harder to detect?
3. List three potentially reversible causes of delirium in advanced cancer.
4. If nonpharmacological or cause-specific strategies to reverse delirium are not successful, what is the best initial medication to treat delirium as a symptom? What dose should you start with?

Depression

1. What are the two best screening questions for depression?
2. When should you consider a psychiatric referral in managing a medically ill patient with depression?
3. If a patient is requesting a hastened death, what questions might you ask to determine if the inquiry is being driven by clinical depression?
4. What are some nonpharmacological techniques that can help with depression?
5. What would be the best acute pharmacological treatment for low-energy depression, especially when the patient may not have a month to wait for SSRIs or TCAs to work? Are there contraindications?

Anxiety

1. Name two nonpharmacological techniques that can help with anxiety.
2. What is the best acute pharmacological treatment for severe anxiety and how would you recommend starting it?

Fatigue

1. What is the difference between primary and secondary fatigue in advanced illness?
2. List three pharmacological approaches to treating fatigue, after you have ruled out reversible secondary causes. What are the main side effects of each?

References

1. American Psychiatric Association. *Diagnostic and Statistical Manual of Mental Disorders*. 5th ed. Washington, DC: American Psychiatric Association; 2013.

2. Hosie A, Davidson PM, Agar M, Sanderson CR, Phillips J. Delirium prevalence, incidence, and implications for screening in specialist palliative care inpatient settings: a systematic review. *Palliat Med*. 2013;27(6):486-498.

3. Spiller JA, Keen JC. Hypoactive delirium: assessing the extent of the problem for inpatient specialist palliative care. *Palliat Med*. 2006;20(1):17-23.

4. White C, McCann MA, Jackson N. First do no harm... Terminal restlessness or drug-induced delirium. *J Palliat Med*. 2007;10(2):345-351.

5. Breitbart W, Alici Y. Agitation and delirium at the end of life: "We couldn't manage him." *JAMA*. 2008;300(24):2898-2910, E2891.

6. Pisani MA, Kong SY, Kasl SV, Murphy TE, Araujo KL, Van Ness PH. Days of delirium are associated with 1-year mortality in an older intensive care unit population. *Am J Respir Crit Care Med*. 2009;180(11):1092-1097.

7. Gusmao-Flores D, Salluh JI, Chalhub RA, Quarantini LC. The Confusion Assessment Method for the Intensive Care Unit (CAM-ICU) and Intensive Care Delirium Screening Checklist (ICDSC) for the diagnosis of delirium: a systematic review and meta-analysis of clinical studies. *Crit Care*. 2012;16(4):R115.

8. Bruera E, Hui D, Dalal S, et al. Parenteral hydration in patients with advanced cancer: a multicenter, double-blind, placebo-controlled randomized trial. *J Clin Oncol*. 2013;31(1):111-118.

9. Irwin SA, Pirrello RD, Hirst JM, Buckholz GT, Ferris FD. Clarifying delirium management: practical, evidenced-based, expert recommendations for clinical practice. *J Palliat Med*. 2013;16(4):423-435.

10. Gagnon B, Low G, Schreier G. Methylphenidate hydrochloride improves cognitive function in patients with advanced cancer and hypoactive delirium: a prospective clinical study. *J Psychiatry Neurosci*. 2005;30(2):100-107.

11. Lo B, Rubenfeld G. Palliative sedation in dying patients: "we turn to it when everything else hasn't worked." *JAMA*. 2005;294(14):1810-1816.

12. Candy B, Jackson KC, Jones L, Leurent B, Tookman A, King M. Drug therapy for delirium in terminally ill adult patients. *Cochrane Database Syst Rev*. 2012;11:CD004770.

13. Rayner L, Loge JH, Wasteson E, Higginson IJ. The detection of depression in palliative care. *Curr Opin Support Palliat Care*. 2009;3(1):55-60.

14. Price A, Hotopf M. The treatment of depression in patients with advanced cancer undergoing palliative care. *Curr Opin Support Palliat Care*. 2009;3(1):61-66.

15. Block SD. Assessing and managing depression in the terminally ill patient. ACP-ASIM End-of-Life Care Consensus Panel. American College of Physicians—American Society of Internal Medicine. *Ann Intern Med*. 2000;132(3):209-218.

16. Miovic M, Block S. Psychiatric disorders in advanced cancer. *Cancer*. 2007;110(8):1665-1676.

17. Ruo B, Rumsfeld JS, Hlatky MA, Liu H, Browner WS, Whooley MA. Depressive symptoms and health-related quality of life: the Heart and Soul Study. *JAMA*. 2003;290(2):215-221.

18. Arroll B, Khin N, Kerse N. Screening for depression in primary care with two verbally asked questions: cross-sectional study. *BMJ*. 2003;327(7424):1144-1146.

19. Chochinov HM, Wilson KG, Enns M, Lander S. Prevalence of depression in the terminally ill: effects of diagnostic criteria and symptom threshold judgments. *Am J Psychiatry*. 1994;151(4):537-540.

20. Fricchione G. Clinical practice. Generalized anxiety disorder. *N Engl J Med*. 2004;351(7):675-682.

21. Horne-Thompson A, Grocke D. The effect of music therapy on anxiety in patients who are terminally ill. *J Palliat Med*. 2008;11(4):582-590.

22. Howard P, Twycross R, Shuster J, Mihalyo M, Wilcock A. Antidepressant drugs. *J Pain Symptom Manage*. 2012;44(5):763-783.

23. Akechi T, Okuyama T, Onishi J, Morita T, Furukawa TA. Psychotherapy for depression among incurable cancer patients. *Cochrane Database Syst Rev*. 2008(2):CD005537.

24. Hardy SE. Methylphenidate for the treatment of depressive symptoms, including fatigue and apathy, in medically ill older adults·and terminally ill adults. *Am J Geriatr Pharmacother*. 2009;7(1):34-59.

25. Candy M, Jones L, Williams R, Tookman A, King M. Psychostimulants for depression. *Cochrane Database Syst Rev*. 2008(2):CD006722.

26. Radbruch L, Strasser F, Elsner F, et al. Fatigue in palliative care patients—an EAPC approach. *Palliat Med*. 2008;22(1):13-32.

27. Yennurajalingam S, Bruera E. Palliative management of fatigue at the close of life: "it feels like my body is just worn out." *JAMA*. 2007;297(3):295-304.

28. Dittner AJ, Wessely SC, Brown RG. The assessment of fatigue: a practical guide for clinicians and researchers. *J Psychosom Res*. 2004;56(2):157-170.

29. Strasser F, Palmer JL, Schover LR, et al. The impact of hypogonadism and autonomic dysfunction on fatigue, emotional function, and sexual desire in male patients with advanced cancer: a pilot study. *Cancer*. 2006;107(12):2949-2957.

30. Del Fabbro E, Garcia JM, Dev R, et al. Testosterone replacement for fatigue in hypogonadal ambulatory males with advanced cancer: a preliminary double-blind placebo-controlled trial. *Support Care Cancer*. 2013;21(9):2599-2607.

31. Payne C, Wiffen PJ, Martin S. Interventions for fatigue and weight loss in adults with advanced progressive illness. *Cochrane Database Syst Rev*. 2012;1:CD008427.

32. Blackhall L, Petroni G, Shu J, Baum L, Farace E. A pilot study evaluating the safety and efficacy of modafinil for cancer-related fatigue. *J Palliat Med*. 2009;12(5):433-439.

33. Bruera E, Strasser F, Shen L, et al. The effect of donepezil on sedation and other symptoms in patients receiving opioids for cancer pain: a pilot study. *J Pain Symptom Manage*. 2003;26(5):1049-1054.

34. Pucci E, Branas P, D'Amico R, Giuliani G, Solari A, Taus C. Amantadine for fatigue in multiple sclerosis. *Cochrane Database Syst Rev*. 2007(1):CD002818.

35. Cruciani RA, Zhang JJ, Manola J, Cella D, Ansari B, Fisch MJ. L-carnitine supplementation for the management of fatigue in patients with cancer: an

eastern cooperative oncology group phase III, randomized, double-blind, placebo-controlled trial. *J Clin Oncol.* 2012;30(31):3864-3869.

36. Tomassini V, Pozzilli C, Onesti E, et al. Comparison of the effects of acetyl L-carnitine and amantadine for the treatment of fatigue in multiple sclerosis: results of a pilot, randomised, double-blind, crossover trial. *J Neurol Sci.* 2004;218(1-2):103-108.

37. Yennurajalingam S, Frisbee-Hume S, Palmer JL, et al. Reduction of cancer-related fatigue with dexamethasone: a double-blind, randomized, placebo-controlled trial in patients with advanced cancer. *J Clin Oncol.* 2013;31(25):3076-3082.

38. Goedendorp MM, Gielissen MF, Verhagen CA, Bleijenberg G. Psychosocial interventions for reducing fatigue during cancer treatment in adults. *Cochrane Database Syst Rev.* 2009(1):CD006953.

SIX

Spiritual and Existential Suffering, the Search for Meaning, and Provider Self-Care

6A | Spiritual and Existential Suffering

Spiritual and existential distress are prevalent in the hospice and palliative care population, though not highly recognized by clinicians. This contrasts with the high importance patients themselves place on spiritual and existential care as part of their overall treatment.[1] Coming to terms with this suffering can be a patient's main task toward the end of life; one of the reasons for optimal control of physical symptoms is to give the patient the presence of mind and precious energy needed for this undertaking.

Once physical symptoms are addressed, spiritual and existential well-being become major determinants of a patient's quality of life and, potentially, his or her quality of death.[1-3] Although it is useful to think of these types of suffering in the discrete categories described below, in reality a patient may experience all or none of the different categories, simultaneously or sequentially.

Spirituality can be defined as the search for meaning and purpose in life and the present moment (transcendence). An individual's spirituality may or may not include belief in God, focus on an afterlife, or membership in a faith community. Spirituality also can be based on humanistic values without inclusion of divinity. Spirituality and religious rituals can be sources of strength for a dying patient. Unaddressed or unresolved spiritual concerns may become immediate and, at times, distressing when a patient faces the prospect of death.

Religions are "belief systems that provide a framework for making sense of life, death, and suffering and responding to universal spiritual questions."[4] They generally involve beliefs, texts, rituals, and other practices that are shared by a community in the context of a relationship with the transcendent.[5] Individuals may have varying levels of religious involvement in their church, synagogue, temple, mosque, or other faith community. Patients who have been extensively involved in their religious faith may find it to be a major source of support during illness; others who have been less involved may find themselves turning toward organized religion during illness; some may feel let down by their religion at this critical time in their lives.

Existential suffering has been viewed as "the distress brought about by the actual or perceived threat to the integrity or continued existence of the whole person."[6] Terminal illnesses can pose a profound threat to an individual's sense of personhood. Cassel identified 14 important aspects of the person, which include personality, past, family, culture, politics, body, and secret life.[7]

Dignity is a word that reflects the ultimate value of a human being.[2] Although dignity is an intrinsic value of human beings, individuals may feel their dignity is threatened when they cannot perform the activities that have provided meaning and purpose throughout their lives (eg, working or caring for others) or when valued physical or mental attributes (eg, independence, cognitive capabilities) are compromised by illness.

Regardless of a patient's spiritual or religious background, the experience of illness and dying can challenge a patient's beliefs, self-perception, and sense of dignity, which can be expressed in multiple ways (**Table 6.1**).

6B | Taking a Spiritual History

Clinicians may wonder whether it is within their role to take a spiritual history. Although it is not likely within their expertise to provide a patient with meaning, value, and reconciliation, it is within a clinician's role to explore the spiritual dimensions of a patient's illness because of the prevalence of spiritual and existential distress among patients, and because of the unique role clinicians have in trying to understand and potentially help alleviate all important dimensions of a patient's

Table 6.1 Expressions of Belief

MEANING	EXPRESSION
Loss of hope	"I don't have a future anymore."
	"I can't see any reason to keep going if I cannot get better."
Loss of meaning	"I can't make any sense out of why this happened to me."
	"How could a caring God allow this to happen to me?"
Loss of value	"I feel I have lost my identity now that I can't work anymore."
	"I feel worthless lying here in bed all the time."
Loss of relationship	"I can't bear the prospect of leaving my family."
	"My sister and I are estranged; I don't know what to say to her."

suffering.[2,3] This has been referred to as *creating an opening* for the patient to express his or her spiritual or existential concerns.[8] Many are reluctant to open up domains that they do not have the expertise to fix, but exploration of these domains demonstrates caring and compassion and lessens the isolation that such suffering can cause for those patients who have no one with whom to share it. This exploration also allows opportunities to facilitate involvement of others with more expertise in these domains, such as a hospital chaplain or someone from the patient's own faith community.

A careful spiritual history can reveal if and how patients' beliefs help or hinder their ability to cope with illness and the prospect of death. Two acronyms have been developed to assist clinicians in remembering the domains that should be explored when taking a spiritual history, FICA[9] and SPIRIT[10] (**Table 6.2**).

Certain questions can be helpful in assessing a patient's spirituality (**Table 6.3**).

Table 6.2 Spiritual History

FICA[9]

F	Faith and beliefs
I	Importance of spirituality in the patient's life
C	(spiritual) Community of support
A	(how does the patient wish spiritual issues to be) Addressed in his or her care

SPIRIT[10]

S	Spiritual belief system
P	Personal spirituality
I	Integration in a spiritual community
R	Ritualized practices and restrictions
I	Implications for medical care
T	Terminal events planning

Table 6.3 Questions to Assess Spirituality

Questions About Hope

As you look to the future, what are your biggest hopes? What about your fears?

Are there things you might hope for even if you cannot be cured?

Does the word "hope" have any spiritual significance for you?

Would anything be left unfinished if you were to die sooner rather than later?

Questions About Meaning

What gives your life the most meaning?

Are there circumstances where your life would not be worth living?

What gives you strength in these difficult times?

Do you have any thoughts about why this happened to you?

If your time were limited, what would be most important to you?

Questions About Values

Are you able to hold on to your sense of dignity and purpose?

What things would be left undone if you were to die sooner rather than later?

How have your family, friends, colleagues, and others been treating you since you became ill?

Are there any spiritual or religious resources you can draw on at this difficult time?

continued

Questions About Relationships

How is your family coping with your illness?

What is it like for you to be taken care of by others after being a caregiver for so long?

Is there anyone you have to make amends with?

How are things between you and God? (Only ask this if the patient is known to be religious.)

6C | The Search for Meaning

Practical Strategies to Enhance Dignity and Meaning

Many strategies address spiritual and existential suffering.[10-12] Some general strategies that can potentially enhance dignity and meaning are within the purview of physicians without specialized training. The more specific strategies generally require special training and may be appropriate and potentially helpful depending on the interests and abilities of the patient, as well as the availability of qualified practitioners. Appropriate members of the interdisciplinary care team can address and offer practical strategies to enhance dignity and meaning for the patient.

General Strategies

The best initial intervention the physician can offer is empathic listening and exploration to ensure that the patient is fully understood. A caring commitment (ie, nonabandonment, supportive counseling by routine caregivers) and response to emotions (ie, acknowledgment, empathy) are the foundations upon which additional focused strategies to enhance dignity and meaning can be employed. The willingness to listen, explore, try to understand, and empathize with patients' spiritual and existential concerns—beginning with the introductory questions outlined above—are core skills for clinicians. Avoid the temptation to be overly reassuring or to try to explain away complex spiritual concerns because it could undermine the opportunity the patient has to feel understood by and connected to the clinician.[2,3] Clinicians must assiduously avoid the temptation to proselytize, prematurely reassure patients, or try to resolve unanswerable questions or events. The lessening of the isolation that stems from sharing these concerns and the willingness to try to help the patient search for an approach that makes sense are key elements of therapeutic strategy. Even if the source of the patient's distress cannot be fixed, the patient no longer is alone—this could be a source of tremendous comfort and a gateway to explore guilt, forgiveness, remorse, and reconciliation in the future. Asking the patient's permission to invite a chaplain or someone from his or her faith tradition to help respond to his or her concerns is an appropriate next step. Palliative care providers should have some familiarity with the end-of-life religious practices that are observed by patients of a specific religion (**Table 6.4**).

Spiritual or Religious Counseling

Referral to a chaplain or clergy from the patient's own religious or spiritual tradition helps those seeking individual religious guidance, spiritual inquiry, or forgiveness or atonement from others or from God.[2,3] Some patients may seek meaning or feel there are redemptive qualities to suffering. Guilt and questioning are common when faced with life-threatening illness.[13] Many patients ask "Why me?" Regardless of the motivations, many people look to their own traditions for answers. Spiritual and religious practices can take on many forms, including prayer, meditation, reading sacred scriptures, and receiving special sacraments or blessings for the sick or dying. These ritual practices can be critical in addressing the spiritual needs of some patients and families. The provider should avoid imposing his or her own religious beliefs and facilitate proper referrals as needed.

Dignity Therapy

Dignity therapy is a therapeutic intervention aimed at alleviating suffering and depression and helping patients find and reshape meaning and dignity.[14] It helps patients address what they find most meaningful and

Table 6.4 Selected End-of-Life Religious Practices for Patients Who Are Dying

RELIGION	END-OF-LIFE PRACTICES
Buddhism	A dying person's state of mind is of great importance; family and friends may repeat mantras to help a patient achieve a peaceful state of mind.
Catholicism	Anointing of the sick, confession, and Holy Communion (requiring a priest) may be a part of end-of-life practices.
Hinduism	Use of prayer beads (mala); strong preference to die at home. Bathing is viewed as both physically and spiritually cleansing and patients may want to be bathed in running water daily.
Islam	Patients may want the opportunity to die facing Mecca; family members may repeat prayers and encourage the patient to repeat the statement of faith.
Judaism	The dying person is encouraged to make a confession, pray for forgiveness, and repeat sacred prayers (Vidui, Shema). Dying patients are attended to constantly, and from the time of death to the funeral, the body is rarely left alone.

identify a personal history they want most remembered. Examples of questions include the following:

- What are your most important accomplishments, and what do you feel most proud of?
- Are there words or perhaps even instructions you would like to offer your family to help prepare them for the future?
- Are there particular things that you feel still need to be said to your loved ones or things that you would want to take the time to say once again?

The answers to such questions can be tape recorded, transcribed, and then provided to the patient as a tangible legacy and permanent record that can be bequeathed to a loved one. Dignity therapy can be provided at the bedside in a relatively short period of time (1- to 2-hour sessions). With such refocusing, some patients truly can find the last phase of life transformational, meaningful, and alive.

A *patient dignity inventory* (PDI) is a reliable instrument for detecting end-of-life-related distress.[15] This 25-item instrument allows patients to evaluate dignity-related themes such as dependency, peace of mind, and self-worth, and can be a useful tool for clinicians to identify a range of issues that may cause distress for patients near the end of life.

Psychotherapy

Psychotherapy programs can be aimed at bolstering adaptive coping mechanisms while minimizing maladaptive mechanisms. For example, meaning-centered group psychotherapy helps patients identify and enhance sources of meaning and purpose in their remaining life.[16] It is provided in a series of group sessions organized around themes with active participation. A patient's ability to participate often depends on prognosis and level of debility as well as the availability of skilled therapists.

Life Review

Having patients actively participate in life review exercises can provide sources of hope and meaning.[17] Such activities focus on strategies to capture a patient's life history. Life review can be therapeutic for patients and can create remembrances for family members left behind. Life review strategies range from simple strategies (eg, reviewing picture albums together) to elaborate ones (eg, creating a series of video messages and remembrances). Other approaches include poems, letters, or presents to be opened at the time of significant future events (eg, graduations, weddings, birth of grandchildren).

Other Specific Interventions

Other specific interventions can be useful depending on patient interest and abilities and available community resources.[18,19] These include music therapy, art therapy, massage, therapeutic touch, humor, distraction, acupuncture, guided imagery, aromatherapy, and biofeedback.

Spirituality and Countertransference

Providers also should have self-awareness and periodic reflection of their own sources of spirituality and meaning.[20] Clinicians must guard against letting their own spiritual and religious beliefs overly influence responses to patients who are in spiritual distress. These encounters can be spiritually enriching, but the patient's spiritual and religious needs always should be addressed first and foremost in this relationship. Although most clinicians who care for seriously ill and dying patients should learn to explore the spiritual dimensions of a patient's illness (if the patient is open to such exploration), the role of trying to resolve the patient's pressing spiritual and religious issues should be left to those with specialized training (chaplains or clergy from the patient's own faith tradition).[2,3]

A patient sometimes will ask the physician to pray with or for him or her. Prayer can be appropriate if it is consistent with the physician's own beliefs and if it is clearly invited by the patient. Physicians who do not feel comfortable in this situation should politely decline and instead offer a chaplain's services. The possibility of prayer together should not be introduced by the physician unless this has been an explicit part of their prior relationship; patients are vulnerable and dependent on physicians at this critical time and may not feel safe declining such offers even if they are uncomfortable.

Healing Presence and Transcendence

Regardless of whether physicians or caregivers have a faith tradition, patients need their caregivers to be a healing presence. Healing sometimes happens when caregivers move beyond objectification and problem solving and instead share the present moment with the patient and family. The healing of loneliness and isolation requires the energy of a nonjudgmental presence, and even love. For a patient facing many uncertainties, it can make a great difference to know that there is a caring presence to accompany them and their family into whatever the future might hold.[20] Rediscovering one's self after being altered by illness often involves the acceptance of help from others; those who have lost parts of themselves can be sustained by another until their own recovery. This is one of the latent functions of physicians—to lend strength and to not abandon the patient no matter how difficult their circumstances may be.[7]

With meticulous physical care, skillful counseling and pastoral care, effective family support, and attentive listening by a concerned person who really cares, physicians can, at times, make it safe enough for a patient to experience transcendence. Transcendence is possibly the most powerful way in which one is restored to wholeness after an injury to personhood. When experienced, transcendence locates the person in a far larger landscape. The sufferer is not isolated by pain, but rather experiences him- or herself as closer to a transpersonal source of meaning and to the human community that shares those meanings. Such an experience need not involve religion in any formal sense; however, in its transpersonal dimension, it is deeply spiritual and intensely human.[7]

6D | Provider Self-Care

Countertransference

It is essential for physicians to be aware of transference and countertransference, especially in the palliative care setting where cases are rife with intense and complex emotions. *Transference* refers to the patient's feelings toward their doctor that may be based on their experiences with other authority figures or others in their lives rather than any particular attributes of the doctor as a person. *Countertransference*, on the other hand, refers to the physician's feelings toward the patient, based more on the physician's personal experience with other patients or significant figures in their lives rather than on the patient as a unique person.

Countertransference can both positively and negatively affect the care the patient receives as well as the emotional life of the physician. On the positive side, countertransference may help with establishing and maintaining an empathic patient-physician relationship (if the patient triggers positive emotions) as well as with prompting physicians to be strong patient advocates. However, more destructive countertransference may emerge if a patient triggers negative emotions, potentially leading the physician to subconsciously avoid particular patients and needed conversations or perhaps give biased advice regarding treatment recommendations and medical decision making. Potential situations that may be influenced by countertransference include

- physician similar to patient with respect to age, profession, personality, or family role
- patient similar to important person in physician's life (mother, father, spouse, children)
- physician fear of particular illnesses and mortality (based on losses and experiences in his or her own family or with prior patients)
- prior personal connection to patient (treating a close friend, colleague, or family member)
- physician is ill or has ill family member or is recently bereaved with unresolved grief.

When a physician notices intense feelings about a case, the first step is to identify the emotion, such as anger, sadness, attraction, dislike, or frustration. Once the reaction is acknowledged, the clinician should explore the origins of the reaction with a close colleague or perhaps a member of the interdisciplinary team. Some reactions can be normalized and legitimized as understandable human responses to complex or tragic situations. Other times, disproportionate reactions that interfere with excellent patient care should be worked through using other methods, such as support groups or therapy. Sometimes other members of the healthcare team who are not experiencing such strong reactions can take on a primary role in the patient's care. Reflecting on such feelings and their potential negative consequences can enable the self-aware physician to attenuate countertransference and still effectively care for the patient.[20]

Provider Burnout

Burnout is defined as a "state of mental and/or physical exhaustion caused by excessive and prolonged stress."[21] Many factors of medical practice can lead physicians to burn out, including work overload, family- and work-life imbalance, insufficient resources, and excessive administrative duties. Physicians also are at risk when they are chronically exposed to the intense suffering experienced by seriously ill patients and their families, especially if they do not have trusted colleagues with whom to explore reactions and challenges. What makes burnout particularly difficult to self-identify and rectify for physicians is that they typically place patients' needs and emotions ahead of their own, potentially leaving their inner lives neither acknowledged nor nurtured. Symptoms are both mental and behavioral, including fatigue, depression, and emotional exhaustion. In addition to the personal toll that burnout inflicts upon physicians, patients and families can be negatively impacted by the impaired performance of their burned-out doctor.

Warning Signs of Burnout

Heightened stress is the first stage of burnout, including
- anxiety, forgetfulness, irritability
- hypertension, bruxism, headaches, palpitations
- insomnia and poor concentration.
  Energy conservation follows:
- increased sleep and work tardiness
- social withdrawal, apathy
- procrastination, inefficiency.

The last stage of burnout is exhaustion, manifested primarily by sadness and departure.[22-24]

Potential Consequences of Burnout

- Neglect of self, family, and social contacts
- Mental illness, substance abuse, suicide
- Reduced productivity and avoidance of engagement with patients and families
- Depersonalization of patients
- Loss of sense of self-worth as a healer
- Increased cynicism and anger[22-25]

How to Avoid or Manage Burnout

There are several ways burnout can be either avoided or addressed. Self-monitoring, often through debriefing with a colleague or other methods of reflection, can help identify rising stress levels early on. The interdisciplinary team, a core part of any palliative care or hospice program, serves a secondary role as an informal arena for clinicians to provide mutual support. A trusted mentor should also be able to help a mentee navigate the challenges of practice as well as steer him or her to available resources, if needed. Finally, more formal mental health services, such as individual psychotherapy, may be necessary to navigate burnout syndrome.

Other methods of self-care include regular exercise, pursuing hobbies, or having a regular spiritual practice.[26] If alcohol or other substance abuse becomes a problem, some states offer confidential treatment programs without negatively impacting professional licensure.[25]

Further Discussion

1. What are the differences between spiritual, religious, and existential suffering?

2. What is dignity and how can it be preserved?

3. What are some general ways that all clinicians can intervene in the face of spiritual, religious, or existential suffering?

4. In addressing and responding to patient suffering, under what circumstances might you request additional help, and where might it come from?

5. Have you had any spiritual or religious issues in your work with patients that made you uncomfortable?

6. What is life review and how may this alleviate existential suffering and help patients find and reshape their dignity?

7. What is one method of taking a spiritual history?

8. What is countertransference?

9. What are some warning signs of clinician burnout?

10. What are some methods or activities to avoid or manage burnout?

References

1. Winkelman WD, Lauderdale K, Balboni MJ, et al. The relationship of spiritual concerns to the quality of life of advanced cancer patients: preliminary findings. *J Palliat Med.* 2011;14(9):1022-1028.

2. Markowitz AJ, McPhee SJ. Spiritual issues in the care of dying patients: ". . . It's okay between me and God." *JAMA.* 2006;296(18):2254.

3. Lo B, Ruston D, Kates LW, et al. Discussing religious and spiritual issues at the end of life: a practical guide for physicians. *JAMA.* 2002;287(6):749-754.

4. Holmes HM, Stein R, Knight CF. *UNIPAC 2. Alleviating Psychological and Spiritual Pain in Patients with Life-Limiting Illness.* 3rd ed. Glenview, IL: American Academy of Hospice and Palliative Medicine; 2008.

5. Sulmasy DP. Spirituality, religion, and clinical care. *Chest.* 2009;135(6):1634-1642.

6. Cassell EJ. Recognizing suffering. *Hastings Cent Rep.* 1991;21(3):24-31.

7. Cassel EJ. The nature of suffering and the goals of medicine. *N Engl J Med.* 1982;306(11):639-645.

8. Boston PH, Mount BM. The caregiver's perspective on existential and spiritual distress in palliative care. *J Pain Symptom Manage.* 2006;32(1):13-26.

9. Puchalski CM. Spirituality and end-of-life care: a time for listening and caring. *J Palliat Med.* 2002;5(2):289-294.

10. Maugans TA. The SPIRITual history. *Arch Fam Med.* 1996;5(1):11-16.

11. Chochinov HM. Dying, dignity, and new horizons in palliative end-of-life care. *CA Cancer J Clin.* 2006;56(2):84-103; quiz 104-105.

12. Chochinov HM, Cann BJ. Interventions to enhance the spiritual aspects of dying. *J Palliat Med.* 2005;8 Suppl 1:S103-115.

13. Sinclair S, Pereira J, Raffin S. A thematic review of the spirituality literature within palliative care. *J Palliat Med.* 2006;9(2):464-479.

14. Chochinov HM, Hack T, Hassard T, Kristjanson LJ, McClement S, Harlos M. Dignity therapy: a novel psychotherapeutic intervention for patients near the end of life. *J Clin Oncol.* 2005;23(24):5520-5525.

15. Chochinov HM, Hassard T, McClement S, et al. The patient dignity inventory: a novel way of measuring dignity-related distress in palliative care. *J Pain Symptom Manage.* 2008;36(6):559-571.

16. Breitbart W. Spirituality and meaning in supportive care: spirituality- and meaning-centered group psychotherapy interventions in advanced cancer. *Support Care Cancer.* 2002;10(4):272-280.

17. Lichter I, Mooney J, Boyd M. Biography as therapy. *Palliat Med.* 1993;7(2):133-137.

18. Herth K. Fostering hope in terminally-ill people. *J Adv Nurs.* 1990;15(11):1250-1259.

19. Freeman L. *A Short Span of Days—Medication and Care for the Dying Patient, Family, and Caregiver.* Ottawa, Canada: Novalis; 1991.

20. Meier DE, Back AL, Morrison RS. The inner life of physicians and care of the seriously ill. *JAMA.* 2001;286(23):3007-3014.

21. Maslach C. *The Cost of Caring*. Englewood Cliffs, NJ: Prentice Hall; 1982.

22. Blust M. Health Professional Burnout: part 1. *Fast Facts and Concepts #167*. Milwaukee, WI: End of Life/Palliative Education Resource Center; 2009. www.eperc.mcw.edu/EPERC/FastFactsIndex/ff_167.htm. Accessed December 15, 2013.

23. Blust M. Health Professional Burnout: part 2. *Fast Facts and Concepts #168*. Milwaukee, WI: End of Life/Palliative Education Resource Center; 2009. www.eperc.mcw.edu/EPERC/FastFactsIndex/ff_168.htm. Accessed December 15, 2013.

24. Blust M. Health Professional Burnout: part 3. *Fast Facts and Concepts #169*. Milwaukee, WI: End of Life/Palliative Education Resource Center; 2009. www.eperc.mcw.edu/EPERC/FastFactsIndex/ff_169.htm. Accessed December 15, 2013.

25. Meier DE, Beresford L. Preventing burnout. *J Palliat Med*. 2006;9(5): 1045-1048.

26. Quill TE, Williamson PR. Healthy approaches to physician stress. *Arch Intern Med*. 1990;150(9):1857-1861.

SEVEN

Goal Setting, Prognosticating, and Surrogate Decision Making

7A | Setting Patient-Centered Goals and Facilitating Transitions

Setting patient-centered goals and facilitating transitions in care are core competencies for palliative care clinicians. The overarching purpose of this communication exchange is to establish goals of current care and anticipate future care needs with patients and families in a process of shared deliberation and decision making.[1-3] Ideally it is a back-and-forth interaction that produces mutual understanding. When done correctly, the quality of medical decisions will improve and trusting relationships will develop. The focus is often assisting with the following discussions and potential decisions:

- risks, benefits, and limitations of disease-directed therapies
- requesting, withholding, or withdrawing therapies
- advance care planning (advance directives and resuscitation preferences)
- hospice selection and timing.

These discussions occur at various points in the course of advancing illness, when patients have emerging symptoms, signs, or test results indicating progressive disease. This information needs to be interpreted in light of the patient's current clinical status, goals, and the available treatment options. The need to renegotiate goals also should be anticipated when triggers of advancing disease suggest limited life expectancy or excessive suffering.[4]

Establishing Patient-Centered Goals

Setting patient-centered goals and facilitating transitions in care includes discussing bad news and incorporating the clinical communication tasks of building rapport, talking about serious news, discussing prognosis, discussing treatment evidence, dealing with conflict, transitioning to end-of-life care, and talking about dying (**Table 7.1**).[1,2,4-7]

Table 7.1 Communicating and Negotiating Goals of Care in Common Palliative Care Settings (Discussing Bad News/Prognosis/Hospice)[1,5-7]	
STEP	
1. Prepare and plan	• Prepare and establish setting. • Identify key stakeholders. • Conduct a premeeting huddle to align the agenda. • Relinquish preset expectations.
2. Find out what the patient and family know and want to know	• Provide sufficient time for patients and families to tell their story; the more patients and families speak early on, the better. • Build relationships and actively listen. • Respect differing preferences about the degree of truth telling.
3. Complete medical review and share information	• Fire a "warning shot." • Discuss prognosis and the benefits and burdens of treatment options. • Be mindful of overly optimistic and overly pessimistic predictions. • Deliver small amounts of information at a time. • Frequently pause to check for understanding.
4. Respond empathetically	• Listen more than talk. • Acknowledge, legitimize, explore, and empathize. • Convey honesty and reframe hope.
5. Identify and resolve conflicts	• Identify potential causes of conflict: information gaps, treatment goal confusion, emotions, family dynamics, team dynamics. • Help resolve conflicts and be prepared to make recommendations. • Recognize that grief work takes time. • Use "I wish" statements.
6. Set goals and plan for future	• Elicit values and preferences. • Establish patient-centered goals. • Be prepared to make a recommendation. • Ask what is most important to the patient. • Summarize goals, establish and implement plan, and follow up.

There are many barriers to effective communication in palliative care, including cultural barriers (ie, lack of experience with death, unrealistic expectations of the healthcare system, cultural beliefs about disclosure of information, trust, family involvement in decision making, filial responsibility), psychological barriers (ie, patient, family, and physician fears), listening barriers, organizational or system barriers, and language barriers. The central theme is knowledge and use of effective communication techniques (**Table 7.2**).[6,8-11]

Table 7.2 Communication Techniques Used in Palliative Care[6,8-11]	
TECHNIQUE	**COMMENT/EXAMPLE**
Build trust.	Encourage patients and families to talk, acknowledge errors, be humble, demonstrate respect, do not force decisions, and listen to what they have to say.
Acknowledge expressed emotions.	"I can see that this is very upsetting." "You seem overwhelmed by this news."
Legitimize the appropriateness and normalcy of the reaction.	"Anyone in your shoes would be upset." "A lot of people would feel angry right now."
Explore more about what is underneath the emotion.	"Tell me what is most upsetting to you." "Tell me what worries you the most."
If you genuinely feel it, empathize.	"I imagine it feels overwhelming." "I would probably feel the same way." "I can't imagine how difficult this is for you."
Explore strengths and coping strategies.	"Where do you find your strength or support?" "In past circumstances, what has helped?"
Use silence effectively.	After delivering bad news, resist the urge to fill silence with more medical facts.
Fire a "warning shot."	"I am afraid I have some difficult news to share with you."

continued

Table 7.2 Communication Techniques Used in Palliative Care[6,8-11] *continued*

TECHNIQUE	COMMENT/EXAMPLE
Pace information and check in periodically.	"Are we on track?" "What haven't we touched upon that is important to you?"
Use the word *dying* effectively.	"Based on what is happening to you and how sick you have become, I believe you are dying."
Be cautious with your use of "I'm sorry."	"I'm sorry" is often misinterpreted as aloofness, pity, or admission of responsibility.
Use "I wish" statements.	Simultaneously express empathy and limits of treatment: "I wish we had better treatments for your condition."
Use communication tools for addressing conflict.	These tools include active listening, explaining your view, reframing, and brainstorming.
Summarize and restate your understanding.	"Let me make sure I understand you correctly."
Provide support.	"We will work through this together." "Is there anyone you would like me to call?"
Recognize and use nonverbal communication.	Ask for clarification when nonverbal communication contradicts a verbal message. Use nonverbal signals that convey empathy.
Use appropriate humor.	When used appropriately, therapeutic humor can build confidence and serve as a way to recognize common dilemmas and paradoxes.

Facilitating transitions and establishing goals of care require leadership in organizing and conducting family meetings with or without the patient present.[5-7] Meeting leadership requires flexibility, patience, group facilitation skills, counseling skills, knowledge of medical and prognostic information, and a willingness to provide guidance in decision making. Family meetings ideally provide a safe environment that is mutually beneficial. Meetings should be proactive when possible and not reactive to crisis situations. They should be offered routinely and conducted at pertinent times thereafter.

Step 1. Prepare and Plan

Initial elements include establishing the proper setting, identifying key stakeholders, and doing your homework. This will include information gathering (ie, collecting medical facts; soliciting opinions from other specialties; and reviewing advance directives, relevant psychosocial data, family dynamics, and known preferences for the handling of medical information) and synthesis. Consider who should be invited and obtain the patient's permission regarding individuals he or she would or would not like to have in attendance. A premeeting huddle with other clinicians who will be present may help you align incentives, anticipate conflicts, and agree upon initial management recommendations. Plan the meeting with an open mind and try to avoid a fixed agenda (eg, to get the do-not-resuscitate order or to stop futile treatment).

Choose an appropriate setting to speak with the patient and family, and when appropriate, use medical interpreters. An environment conducive to effective communication should be quiet, private, and include adequate seating. If the patient lacks capacity, ask if the family would be more comfortable meeting outside the patient's room. A box of facial tissues should be available. Allot adequate time and ensure that interruptions are kept to a minimum by arranging to hold or silence mobile phones and pagers.

Step 2. Find Out What the Patient and Family Know and Want to Know

The early steps of the discussion are important for a successful meeting. Begin with introductions of those in attendance and a statement of the goals for the meeting. Ask the patient and family if they agree with the agenda and if other items should be addressed. If you can only commit a certain amount of time, let the attendees know the time constraints so they will not feel abruptly cut short. If you do not know the patient or family well, spend some time building a relationship and establishing trust. Allow patients and families sufficient time to tell their stories. In general, the more patients and families speak in the early parts of such meetings, the better.

Establish how much the patient knows and wants to know. Always invite the patient or family to provide their understanding of medical information. Questions might include

- Can you describe for me your sense of how things are going?
- What have the doctors told you about your condition?
- How have things been going for you over the past several months?

Some patients may want to know very little; others may want as much detail as possible. Still other patients may not be capable of understanding medical information or may designate someone else to communicate on their behalf. In these cases, ask the patient and family how they would like to receive information. Possible questions include

- Would you like me to tell you the full details of your condition?
- Some people really do not want to be told what is wrong with them but would rather their families be told instead. What do you prefer?

Step 3. Medical Review—Sharing Information

After you have heard what the patient or family knows, you can confirm their understanding, provide new information, and clarify or correct potential misunderstandings. Asking the patient's permission to bring them up to date is courteous and focuses attention on what will follow. Cultural norms and patient preferences on the degree of truth telling should be respected. Whenever possible, the clinician most closely aligned with the patient's ongoing treatment should participate in and begin the discussion.

The provider then needs to share the relevant information (eg, results of studies, status of the disease, or prognosis, depending on the starting point of the discussion). When potentially life-altering information needs to be shared, these are often experienced as bad news discussions.[12] "Firing a warning shot" to alert the patient or family of impending bad news is a useful initial communication strategy; for example, "I am afraid I have some difficult news to share with you."

The amount of information should be paced with frequent pauses to allow time for affective responses (eg, anger, fear, relief, regret). Use silence and body language as tools to facilitate the discussion. Let the patient process the information, and resist the urge to fill the silence with more facts. Move the conversation forward one step at a time. Check in periodically, making sure the discussion is in keeping with the patient's needs:

- Are we on track?
- What haven't we touched upon that is important to you?

Avoid medical jargon and provide succinct summaries of the current situation, focusing on issues of most importance to patients (ie, function/quality/time). On one hand, the clinician should not minimize the severity of the situation; on the other, information should be delivered in an honest, straightforward, and caring manner that is not too blunt. For example:

- The worsening weakness and shortness of breath you describe is from the cancer, which is growing despite our best efforts.
- I know that your appetite is down and you are not able to get around much anymore; unfortunately, your heart disease is getting worse despite our best treatments.

If the patient is likely to die within days, weeks, or even months, it is appropriate to use the word *dying* in the conversation: "Based on what is happening to you and how sick you have become, I believe you are dying."

Well-intentioned efforts to soften the blow may lead to vagueness and confusion, making subsequent conversations more difficult.

Step 4. After the News—Responding Empathetically

The skilled clinician flexibly assesses, probes, and paces the content and depth of the discussions and negotiations in an emotionally responsive and culturally competent manner. Try to balance emotional support with informational needs. Patients and families respond to bad news in a variety of ways: affective (tears, anger, anxiety, fear), cognitive (denial, blame, guilt, disbelief), spiritual (Why me?), or somatic (numbness, disorientation, fight or flight response). Rather than immediately trying to limit emotion, give the patient and family time to react and to express their immediate feelings. Be prepared to support them through a broad range of reactions using communication techniques described in Table 7.2. "I wish" statements are often useful because they can simultaneously express empathy while at the same time emphasize the limits on medical interventions[9]:

- I wish we had better treatments for your condition.
- I wish things were different.

Use "I'm sorry" statements cautiously. Although they may communicate empathy and sorrow, they can be misinterpreted as pity, aloofness, or admission of responsibility. Nonverbal communication may also be very helpful. Consider touching the patient in an appropriate, reassuring manner.

Step 5. Identify and Resolve Conflicts

After emotions have been acknowledged and processed, the conversation may proceed in one of two directions: acceptance or nonacceptance. If the patient and family accept the information, several types of questions usually follow:

- How long?
- What will happen?
- Will I suffer?
- What do we do now?

When patients and family are ready to move on and discuss next steps, the conversation can move on to setting goals and planning for the future.

At times, patients and family members are not prepared to accept the information and the limits of medical treatment.[11,13] Questions or statements that might arise include

- We are not giving up—we want everything done!
- There must be some mistake!
- There must be something you can do!
- We believe in miracles. She is a fighter and will never give up.

In the setting of nonacceptance or denial, identify, try to understand, and eventually help resolve conflicts among patients, family members, and providers. Conflicts can arise between the patient and clinician, family and clinician, clinicians, and family members.

These conflicts often arise from subtle differences in how key stakeholders interpret risks and benefits of treatment based on affective, cognitive, spiritual, or family concerns. Reasons for communication breakdowns around end-of-life decision making include (a) information that is inaccurate, inconsistent, confusing, excessive, or genuinely uncertain; (b) unclear treatment goals or differing priorities; (c) emotions such as grief, fear, guilt, or anger; (d) dysfunctional family system or consulting teams that disagree about best approach; and (e) mistrust or genuine value differences between the clinician and the patient or surrogate.

When confronted with a conflict, do not avoid or deny it. Get the facts straight and try to understand the patient's or family's goals. Do not fight or argue over the facts. Respond to emotions. Remember that grief work takes time, and be prepared to support the patient and family using other members of the interdisciplinary team (ie, chaplain, social services, ethics consultant). Allow expressions of hope even if they are unrealistic. Rather than reiterating what medicine cannot do, use "I wish" statements to gently reframe hope on more realistic goals. Try to find common ground, be creative with solutions, and judiciously use time-limited trials when appropriate.[14] Try not to be defensive or argumentative.

Step 6. Set Goals and Plan for the Future

The prior steps are designed to lead to a discussion of patient-centered goals in light of a common understanding of the patient's new reality. A useful way of starting a goal-setting conversation is by saying, "We have discussed your condition and the reality that time may be short. With that in mind, what is most important to you? What do you need to accomplish? Who do you need to see in case time is shorter than we hope?"

After each question, the patient should be given sufficient time to answer. Use probing follow-up questions if necessary and react appropriately to affective responses (Table 7.2). Discuss big picture goals before exploring specific interventions. Common patient-centered goals often incorporate elements of family, home, relationships, dignity, and comfort. After the patient has had time to articulate his or her goals, restate them to be sure you fully understand; for example, "What I hear you saying is that you want to be home, comfortable, and survive until your daughter gives birth so you can meet your grandchild."

When the goals have been established, providers should review the patient's current medical treatments (ie, medications, tests, monitoring) and potential planned interventions (ie, CPR, intubation, dialysis, hospitalization) and decide which will help the patient achieve his or her goals based on treatment philosophy and clinical condition. As a general rule, discuss what you can do before discussing what you cannot do. Those current or future treatment options that would not help achieve the patient's goals should be discussed for potential discontinuation. There is no need to ask about every single treatment. The clinician should be prepared to make recommendations or propose a treatment philosophy based on what is known about the patient's medical condition and their goals, values, and preferences[11]; for example, "Based on where you are in your illness, and what I am hearing you say is most important to you, I'm not sure it makes sense to (stay in the hospital, finish your antibiotics, consider dialysis, consider resuscitation if your heart stops, etc.). What do you think?"

If the patient's goals are unrealistic (surviving to a specific improbable date, belief in miracles), it is important to say so using strategies to preserve and potentially reframe hope, including ways to hope for the best while simultaneously preparing for the worst.[9] If there is disagreement about how a particular treatment might meet the patient's goals, or genuine uncertainty regarding the prognosis, a time-limited treatment trial might be considered. Commitments to minimize suffering, to not abandon the patient and family, and to appropriately refer for emotional and practical support (eg, family, significant others, friends, social worker, spiritual counselor, peer support group, professional therapist, hospice, home health agency) are essential. At the end of the discussions, the provider should summarize key aspects of agreed-upon next steps, invite questions, and close the meeting.

Special Considerations

Managing Uncertainty

Uncertainty is the rule in palliative care, and most patients want physicians to acknowledge that prognosis is uncertain.[15] Confronting uncertainty takes time, confidence, and emotional energy. The acknowledgment of uncertainty, however, must simultaneously be countered with a commitment to a meaningful engagement and nonabandonment during the course of one's illness. It also requires that clinicians give patients and families signposts that they can use to understand if things are getting better or worse. The challenge is to offer patients and families the ability to simultaneously hope for the best and prepare for the worst.[10] Another approach to managing uncertainty is the use of time-limited trials, which is an agreement between the patient, his or her family, and clinicians to use certain medical therapies over a defined period to assess the patient's response according to previously agreed upon clinical outcomes that define relative successes or failures in view of the patient's goals.[16] A time-limited trial allows opportunity for evaluation of trends and progress, patient reflection, family input, goals setting, adaptation to a new normal, palliation of symptoms and suffering, building trust, recruiting community resources, and rehabilitation and functional improvement.

Cultural Competence

Cultural competence means making every effort to respect cultural diversity and to explore and understand the different cultural norms that each patient and family brings to end-of-life encounters based on their background, ethnicity, and upbringing.[8] Although there is no one-size-fits-all approach, cultural competence involves recognizing one's own cultural biases and understanding each patient's and family's preference for information sharing and decision making. This often includes respecting different degrees of truth telling, recognizing preferences for patient-centered versus family-centered styles of decision making, as well as preferences for more paternalistic or collaborative styles to inform choice. Failure to recognize and incorporate these dynamics into the communication approach will lead to misunderstanding, increased conflict, and poor decisions.

For example, most patients want to be fully informed of their diagnosis and prognosis. There are some cultures, however, where disclosure of truth is believed to cause bad outcomes (eg, traditional Navajo cultures), and nondisclosure is seen as protective and benevolent (eg, Bosnian immigrants). There are even some cultures in which patients want to know the truth but want to learn it through nonverbal means or by inference (eg, some Asian cultures, Japanese-speaking Americans). Therefore, clinicians must respect the type of information patients and families seek, their desires for information sharing, and the cultural norms they bring to each clinical encounter. Open-ended questions that can begin to explore these preferences include

- How do people from your culture (country, community, etc.) talk about illness?
- If we don't tell your father his diagnosis, how should we share important information and how do we make decisions about his treatment?

The key to improving cultural competence and preventing misunderstanding is through self-awareness and education. Outreach programs to minority groups have also proved very effective.[17] One also should recognize that there is considerable variation within groups, so culturally based preferences should never be assumed. For example, many Japanese Americans' preferences have shifted to a more traditionally Western style, including an increased desire for full disclosure and decreased desire of disclosure through only nonverbal means.

When Patients and Families Want "Everything"

Considerable conflicts sometimes exist (Step 5) when patients and families want "everything."[13] Providers should not take this statement at face value. Rather, this statement needs a full exploration to identify the treatment philosophy underlying the request. For example, the request may range from everything that might provide maximum relief of suffering even if it might unintentionally shorten life to everything that has any potential to prolong life even a small amount. Potential thoughts underlying requests for "everything" include fear of dying, fear of abandonment, wanting reassurances that all options have been exhausted, faith in God's will, and family conflicts about different values and perceptions (Table 7.3). When requests for burdensome treatments that are very unlikely to work persist, the provider should honor the request so that the patient and family feel heard and respected (eg, writing a "full CPR—no limits" order). However, under these circumstances, providers should also consider a series of harm-reduction strategies, including (a) stop regularly discussing limitations on burdensome interventions unless brought up by the family, (b) address the medical team's discomfort and disapproval by communicating with them the reasoning behind the decision and by finding other goals to work on (symptom relief, emotional support), and (c) use clinical judgment to limit burdensome treatments that do not advance the patient's goals. This latter strategy might include initiating CPR but limiting to only one or two cycles if the patient does not respond, which simultaneously addresses the patient's and family's concern that everything was done, but limits the burden of a futile procedure.

Table 7.3 Potential Underlying Meanings of "Everything"

DOMAIN	CONCEPT	WHAT "EVERYTHING" MEANS	QUESTIONS TO ASK
Affective	Abandonment	"Don't give up on me."	"What worries you the most?"
	Fear	"Keep trying for me."	
	Anxiety	"I don't want to leave my family."	"What are you most afraid of?"
	Depression	"I'm scared of dying."	"What does your doctor say about your prospects?"
		"I would feel like I'm giving up."	"What is the hardest part for you?"
			"What are you hoping for?"

continued

Table 7.3 Potential Underlying Meanings of "Everything" *continued*

DOMAIN	CONCEPT	WHAT "EVERYTHING" MEANS	QUESTIONS TO ASK
Cognitive	Incomplete understanding	"I do not really understand how sick I am."	"What are your most important goals?"
	Seeking reassurance that best medical care has been given	"Do everything you think is worthwhile." "Don't leave any stone unturned."	"What is your understanding of your condition and prognosis?" "What have others told you about what is going on with your illness?"
	Seeking reassurance that all possible life-prolonging treatment is given	"I really want every possible treatment that has a chance of helping me live longer." "I will go through anything, regardless of how hard it is."	"What have they said the impact of these treatments would be?" "Tell me more about what you mean by 'everything.'"
Spiritual	Vitalism	"I value every moment of life, regardless of the pain and suffering, which has important meaning for me."	"Does your religion (faith) provide any guidance in these matters?"
	Faith in God's will	"I will leave my fate in God's hands; I am hoping for a miracle; only He can decide when it is time to stop."	"How might we know when God thinks it is your time?"
Family	Differing perceptions	"I cannot bear the thought of leaving my children (wife/husband)."	"How is your family handling this?"
	Family conflict	"My husband will never let me go."	"What do your children know?"
	Children or dependents	"My family is only after my money." "I don't want to bother my children with all of this."	"Have you made plans for your children or other dependents?" "Have you discussed who will make decisions for you if you cannot?" "Have you completed a will?"

From Quill TE, Arnold R, Back AL. Discussing treatment preferences with patients who want "Everything." Ann Intern Med. 2009;151:345-349.13 ©2009 American College of Physicians. All rights reserved. Adapted with permission.

Introducing Hospice

The initial exploration of hospice often requires discussing bad news.[18] Patients and families who have invested time, energy, and meaning in disease-directed medical treatment have to be told that treatment is no longer effective, that they are likely to die in the next 6 months, and that the only treatments they will receive while on hospice will be palliative. Although hospice has many benefits (see chapter 1), the information about lack of effective treatment for their disease and about limited prognosis is emotionally laden and can sometimes be hard for patients to accept. Some patients and families may have had prior positive or negative experiences with hospice care, or they may hold preconceived ideas regarding how hospice care is delivered. This can strongly influence their perspectives on hospice discussions. The same six-step process for facilitating transitions and setting goals is a way to initiate the hospice discussion, to deal with affective responses, and to explore the risks and benefits of the various options for continuing treatment. Many patients require several visits to accept this transition and may need to explore second opinions about available experimental treatment alternatives before accepting hospice. Although fewer patients are dying in hospitals, there is still an increasing use of the intensive care unit in the last month of life.[19] Nationwide, approximately 45% of patients who die are admitted to hospice and many of those are for hours or days (the median hospice stay is about 19 days),[20] which is indicative of how hard this transition is for patients and families and how important it is for clinicians to use the techniques described in this chapter.

7B | Estimating and Communicating Prognosis

A core component of information shared in the palliative care setting is estimating and communicating prognosis. Prognosis is a prediction of likely future outcomes of a disease (ie, survival, symptoms, function, quality of life, family impact, financial concerns) with or without treatment.[21,22] Understanding prognosis is central to establishing patient-centered goals and making decisions about disease-directed treatment as well as hospice. In the palliative care setting, prognosis is one of the main elements of discussion when talking about serious news and establishing goals of care.

Inaccurate predictions of prognosis may lead to poor decision making. Overly optimistic predictions can lead to overuse of ineffective or unwanted disease-directed treatment, delay in hospice referrals, false hope, unrealistic expectations, unnecessary tests and procedures, and poor symptom control. At the time of hospice referral, physicians tend to overestimate survival in patients with advanced cancer by about 30%, and the bias is more pronounced the longer the physician-patient relationship.[23] Overly pessimistic predictions can lead to underuse of treatments and life-sustaining interventions, resulting in shortened survival and premature deaths.[24] Therefore, accurately estimating and communicating prognosis are central to high-quality decision making in advanced disease and at the end of life.[25]

Estimating Prognosis

We recommend a structured approach to formulating a prediction, including anticipating the type of prognostic information most likely needed during the discussion and anchoring the disease course on the most likely disease trajectory (see Figure 1.1 [p. 5]).[26,27] Then the prognosis is tailored to the individual patient based on the best available evidence. There are many sources of data that can be used to assist with prognostication in palliative care.[21,28] These include functional status scales, signs and symptoms, physiological variables, disease-based prediction rules, Web-based programs, and hospice eligibility criteria (**Table 7.4**). Prior studies have assessed the accuracy of clinicians' subjective prediction of survival. However, with accumulating information about prognosis and the widely accepted value of evidence-based medicine, clinicians' prognostic judgments should always be supported by the best available data, appropriately selected from the sources below. For each of these information sources, the provider needs to perform an evidence-based appraisal of the validity and reliability of the prognostic data, as well as their applicability to the particular patient (eg, similar in age, disease stage, comorbidities), setting (eg, outpatient, hospital-based, hospice enrollee), protective factors, and willingness to live.[29] One also

Table 7.4 Sources of Prognostic Information in Palliative Care

SOURCE	SCALE/PROGNOSTIC MODEL/ DISEASE	COMMENTS
Functional status scales	Palliative Performance Scale Palliative Prognostic Index Palliative Prognostic Score	These scales allow for rapid estimates of life expectancy that place patients in groupings that differ significantly in survival. They also take advantage of the fact that patients who are terminally ill have a convergence of symptoms as the time of their death nears.
Signs, symptoms, and physiological variables	Advanced cancer—anorexia-cachexia syndrome, dyspnea, delirium, certain physiological variables Hypoxic ischemic encephalopathy—absent pupillary or corneal reflex at Day 3	The strength of these individual correlations is rarely sufficient enough to rely upon solely when prognosticating with patients and families. One exception to this rule is absent pupillary and corneal reflexes on Day 3 in patients with hypoxic ischemic encephalopathy.
Generic, organ-specific, disease-based prediction rules	Generic—APACHE II, III, IV; SAPS II, III Organ-specific—multiple organ dysfunction score Disease-based—Glasgow coma scale, ICH Score, Takuhashi scoring system for metastatic spinal tumors	Many prognostication systems and prediction rules exist, but all should be used with caution for individual predictions and decision making.
Web-based prognostic tools	Palliative care patients—Prognosat Elderly patients—ePrognosis Heart failure—Seattle Heart Failure Model Head injury prognosis—CRASH model	A growing number of Web-based prognostic tools are available. As with the other information sources, use caution when accessing these tools for individual predictions and decision making.
Hospice eligibility criteria	Amyotrophic lateral sclerosis, cancer, cardiovascular disease, end-stage dementia, HIV, liver disease, multiple sclerosis, Parkinson's disease, pulmonary disease, stroke, and coma	Hospice guidelines do not represent hard and fast requirements. The eligibility guideline may also vary with the Medicare fiscal intermediary.

should be aware of the potential personal, system-level, and emotional factors that may bias one's prediction and the potential strategies to overcome these influences when communicating the information.

Functional Status Scales

A number of easy-to-use scales and indices have been developed to permit rapid estimates of life expectancy, placing patients in groupings that differ significantly in survival. These scales include the Palliative Performance Scale (PPS) (**Table 7.5**), the Palliative Prognostic Index (PPI), the Palliative Prognostic Score (PaP), and the Karnofsky Performance Scale (KPS), among others. These scales take advantage of the fact that patients who are terminally ill, regardless of the diagnosis, have a convergence of symptoms as the time of their death approaches. In advanced illnesses, common symptoms known to be predictive of short-term survival (ie, less than 6 months) include ambulatory status, performance status, nutritional intake, and mental status. For example, the PPS is a simple measure that incorporates these dimensions on a 100-point scale (100% = normal, 0% = dead) in 10-point increments (Table 7.5).[30] On an initial consult to a palliative care service, PPS scores of 10%, 20%, 30%, 40%–60%, and ≥70% provide distinct survival curves, which can be helpful in decision making (**Figure 7.1**).[31]

Table 7.5 Palliative Performance Scale, Version 2 (PPSv2)

PPS	AMBULATION	ACTIVITY AND EVIDENCE OF DISEASE	SELF-CARE	INTAKE	CONSCIOUS LEVEL
100%	Full	Normal activity and work No evidence of disease	Full	Normal	Full
90%	Full	Normal activity and work No evidence of disease	Full	Normal	Full
80%	Full	Normal activity with effort Some evidence of disease	Full	Normal or reduced	Full
70%	Reduced	Unable to do normal job/work Significant disease	Full	Normal or reduced	Full
60%	Reduced	Unable to do hobby/house work Significant disease	Occasional assistance necessary	Normal or reduced	Full or confusion
50%	Mainly sit/lie	Unable to do any work Extensive disease	Considerable assistance required	Normal or reduced	Full or confusion
40%	Mainly in bed	Unable to do most activity Extensive disease	Mainly assistance	Normal or reduced	Full or drowsy +/- confusion
30%	Totally bed bound	Unable to do any activity Extensive disease	Total care	Normal or reduced	Full or drowsy +/- confusion
20%	Totally bed bound	Unable to do any activity Extensive disease	Total care	Minimal to sips	Full or drowsy +/- confusion
10%	Totally bed bound	Unable to do any activity Extensive disease	Total care	Mouth care only	Full or drowsy +/- confusion
0%	Death	-	-	-	-

continued

Table 7.5 Palliative Performance Scale, Version 2 (PPSv2) *continued*

Instructions for Use of PPS

1. PPS scores are determined by reading horizontally at each level to find a best fit for the patient, which is then assigned as the PPS % score.

2. Begin at the left column and read downwards until the appropriate ambulation level is reached, then read directly across to the next column and downwards again until the activity/evidence of disease is located. Do not go upward in the columns as you move to the right. These steps are repeated until all five columns are covered before assigning the actual PPS for that patient. In this way, leftward columns (columns to the left of any specific column) are stronger determinants and generally take precedence over others.

   Example 1: A patient who spends the majority of the day sitting or lying down due to fatigue from advanced disease and requires considerable assistance to walk, even for short distances, but who is otherwise fully conscious with good intake, would be scored at PPS 50%.

   Example 2: A patient who has become paralyzed and quadriplegic requiring total care would be PPS 30%. Although this patient may be placed in a wheelchair (and perhaps seem initially to be at 50%), the score is 30% because he or she would be otherwise totally bed bound due to the disease or complication if it were not for caregivers providing total care, including lift and transfer. The patient may have normal intake and full conscious level.

   Example 3: However, if the patient in example 2 was paraplegic and bed bound but still able to do some self-care such as feed himself, then the PPS would be higher at 40% or 50% because he or she is not "total care."

3. PPS scores are in 10% increments only. Sometimes there are several columns easily placed at one level but one or two that seem better at a higher or lower level; however, choosing a "halfway" value of PPS 45% is not correct. The combination of clinical judgment and "leftward precedence" is used to determine whether 40% or 50% is the more accurate score for that patient.

4. PPS may be used for several purposes. First, it is an excellent communication tool for quickly describing a patient's current functional level. Second, it may have value in criteria for workload assessment or other measurements and comparisons. Finally, it appears to have prognostic value.

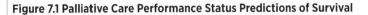

Figure 7.1 Palliative Care Performance Status Predictions of Survival

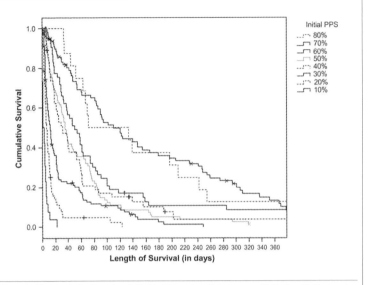

Initial PPS
- 80%
- 70%
- 60%
- 50%
- 40%
- 30%
- 20%
- 10%

Adapted with permission from Lau F, Maida V, Downing M, Lesperance M, Karlson N, Kuziemsky C. Use of the Palliative Performance Scale (PPS) for end-of-life prognostication in a palliative medicine consultation service. J Pain Symptom Manage. 2009;37(6):969. ©2009 Elsevier. All rights reserved.

Individual Signs, Symptoms, and Physiological Variables

The presence of individual signs, symptoms, and physiological variables can also correlate with survival.[32,33] In advanced cancer, for example, anorexia-cachexia syndrome, dyspnea, delirium, and certain biological variables (eg, hypoalbuminemia, leukocytosis, lymphocytopenia, C-reactive protein) have all been shown to correlate with survival. The strength of these individual correlations, however, is rarely sufficiently high enough to rely upon solely when prognosticating with patients and families. The one possible exception is for patients with severe hypoxic ischemic encephalopathy after a cardiac arrest. For these patients, the absence of pupillary light or corneal reflexes on Day 3 uniformly predicts a poor prognosis, defined as death or severe disability.[32]

Generic, Organ-Specific, Disease-Based Prognostication Systems and Prediction Rules

Many models exist to assist with prognostic estimates, including those designed to measure severity of disease for adults admitted to the intensive care unit (eg, APACHE II, III, IV; SAPS III, III), organ-dysfunction prognostic models (eg, sepsis-related organ failure score, multiple organ dysfunction score), as well as disease-specific prediction-rules models (eg, head injury, cancer, liver disease, intracerebral hemorrhage, spinal cord compression, hypoxic ischemic injury after cardiac arrest).[24,34-39] Many of these models take into account patient characteristics, disease characteristics, and physiological variables. The most important limiting factor is the lack of individual prognostic ability, as most of these prognostication systems and prediction rules were not designed for individualized decision making. Therefore, they should be used with extreme caution in such a context.

Web-Based Prediction Rules

There are a number of Web-based prognostic tools that are now available for palliative care patients and for patients with cancer, head injury, and heart failure. Prognostat (https://htg.his.uvic.ca/tools/PrognosticTools/PalliativePerformanceScale/Prognostat/index.php) is an interactive prognostic tool used to estimate chances of survival for palliative care patients based on gender, age, diagnosis, and initial PPS score.[40] ePrognosis (http://eprognosis.ucsf.edu) is an interactive prognostic tool for elderly patients that provides 1-year mortality estimates based on patients with similar demographic and comorbid conditions.[41] The Seattle Heart Failure Model website (http://depts.washington.edu/shfm) provides a calculator of projected survival at baseline and after interventions for patients with congestive heart failure.[42] Finally, the CRASH Head Injury Prognosis model (www.crash.lshtm.ac.uk/Risk%20calculator) is used as an aid to estimate mortality at 14 days and death and severe disability at 6 months in patients with traumatic brain injury.[43]

Hospice Determination of Prognosis

Hospice eligibility is based on the patient's proximity to the end of life and is determined by a comprehensive assessment of the patient, family, and disease course. Hospice medical directors must determine if there are clinical indicators of advancing disease, if they would be surprised if the patient died in the next 6 months, and whether the patient and family have made a clear choice for comfort care only.[44]

Individualized Prognostication

Each patient should have an individualized prognosis. In developing a patient-specific prognosis, it is useful to start with a generalized prognosis based on a subjective assessment and knowledge of disease trajectories. Knowledge of disease trajectories is important because predictions are easier and more accurate in the short period of evident decline trajectory compared with the re-entry, dwindling, and sudden neurological impairment trajectory (see chapter 1). Once you have formulated a general prognosis, the estimate should then be modified based on a critical appraisal of the literature and the particulars of the patient, including signs, symptoms, comorbidities, and the patient's desire to continue to pursue disease-directed therapy.

Communicating Prognosis

After you have formulated your best prognostic estimate, the key prognostic message should be coordinated across the care team to avoid confusion and providing mixed messages to the patient and family. When communicating prognosis, similar principles and recommendations apply to the structured approach as to when you are setting patient-centered goals and facilitating transitions in care: (1) prepare and plan, (2) find out what the patient and family know and want to know, (3) share information from medical review, (4) respond empathetically after the news, (5) identify and resolve conflicts, and (6) set goals and plan for the future.

You should assess the desire and readiness of the patient for prognostic information. Eighty percent of patients and families want to know prognosis; they both dread and crave it. However, about 20% of patients and families may prefer not to know their complete prognostic information or may want it communicated in a particular way. **Figure 7.2** provides an approach for patients and families who (a) want to know prognosis, (b) do not want to know prognosis, or (c) are ambivalent and afraid of finding out the information.[45]

For individual prognostication, considerable uncertainty remains the rule. Therefore, it is important to integrate both evidence- and experience-based medicine and present the information in formats tailored to the particular patient. Prognostic estimates should be bounded with ranges of time to convey realistic uncertainty, being sure to allow for exceptions in both optimistic and pessimistic directions. One example of how the prognostic message can be delivered is by using the following caveat-ballpark-exceptions format:

- Caveat
  - It is impossible to predict for any individual with certainty, but...
- Ballpark
  - the average person with your illness will live [hours to days, days to weeks, few weeks to a few months, several months] and...
  - treatment, if it works, might extend that time [a month or two].
- Exceptions
  - It could be longer, and we will do everything in our power to give you as much time as possible.
  - Unfortunately, it could also be shorter, so we better get prepared just in case.

For survival-predominant prognoses (eg, "How long do I have?"), be mindful of overly optimistic prognoses, and remember to always include exceptions in both directions (eg, "Some may live longer, but others may unfortunately live less time."). For outcome-predominant prognoses (eg, "What will life be like?"), be mindful of overly pessimistic predictions by remembering the power of adaptation and engendering hope by helping patients and families find new meaning.

When discussing treatment benefits, be aware that relative expressions of benefit (ie, a 10% relative risk reduction when describing a treatment that reduces the risk of a bad outcome from 10% to 9%) may exaggerate treatment benefits compared to absolute expressions (ie,

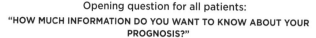

Figure 7.2 Patient-Centered Communication When Discussing Prognosis

Opening question for all patients:

"HOW MUCH INFORMATION DO YOU WANT TO KNOW ABOUT YOUR PROGNOSIS?"

Patient wants to know about prognosis	Patient does not want to know about prognosis	Patient is ambivalent or very afraid about knowing prognosis
Determine the specific information the patient wants to know and how the patient wants it to be presented.	Assess why the patient prefers not to talk about the prognosis (eg, "Could you help me understand why you do not want to discuss your prognosis?").	Acknowledge the patient's ambivalence (eg, "It sounds like you are having difficulty deciding if you want to know this information; is that correct?").
Provide the information using the "caveat-ballpark-exception" format (eg, "It is impossible to predict for any individual with certainty, but the average person with your illness will usually live a month or 2. It could be longer but it could also be shorter.").	Verbally acknowledge the patient's informational and emotional concerns; use empathic statements (eg, "I understand this may be difficult for you to discuss.").	Explore the patient's underlying concern of knowing versus not knowing the prognosis.
Verbally acknowledge the patient's reaction; use empathic statements.	If the patient needs to know the prognosis to make important decisions, consider providing limited information or asking the patient to designate a proxy to receive the information.	Verbally acknowledge and legitimize the patient's reaction; use empathic statements.
Assess the patient's understanding of the information presented (eg, "Could you tell me what we discussed today?").		Provide options for how the information can be presented.

Adapted with permission from Ngo-Metzger Q, August KJ, Srinivasan M, Liao S, Meyskens Jr, FL. End-of-life care: guidelines for patient-centered communication. Am Fam Physician. *2008; 77(2):167-174.*

a 1% absolute risk reduction when describing a treatment that reduces the risk of a bad outcome from 10% to 9%). Also, given the known effects of framing bias, information should be presented in both a positive frame (eg, "She has a 30% chance of surviving.") as well as a negative frame (eg, "She has a 70% chance of dying."). People also interpret probabilities (10% chance) and proportions (1 out of 10 chances) differently and respond to graphical presentations of data differently than spoken numerical presentations. Clinicians need to hone their skills to communicate treatment evidence using a variety of techniques and be able to adjust to different settings and learning styles of patients and families.

Be honest and engender hope—not the kind of hope that pivots on cures or physical improvements, but the kind of hope that helps people adapt and find new meaning and valued life activities. Finally, when in doubt, insert a time-limited trial; a few extra days or weeks of observance may improve your prognostic estimates, help resolve lingering conflicts, and allow additional time for the necessary grief work to occur.

7C | Surrogate Decision Making and Working with Families

Because many patients in palliative care lack capacity, provider skills in working with families and surrogate decision makers are essential.[46,47] Surrogate decision making can be informed by a hierarchy of information from advance directives, substituted judgment, or best interests.[48] End-of-life decision making is often dynamic, and all sources of information should be drawn from so that the patient's voice is brought into the center of the decision-making process (ie, "If mom were here sitting with us, what would she say?" "In light of what we have talked about so far, what do you think dad would want to do?").

Although surrogate decision makers do not perfectly predict patient treatment preferences, they provide insight into a patient's prior values.[49] Surrogate decision makers rarely rely solely on the physician's estimate of prognosis and estimate their own prognosis from a variety of sources—and this may be a source of conflict that needs exploration.[50]

And just like patients, surrogate decision makers often are overly optimistic in predicting their loved one's prognosis.[51]

Family members should not feel alone in making medical decisions, and providers need to be aware of the intense emotional burden felt by up to one-third of surrogate decision makers that can persist long after decisions are made.[52] As a result, grief and bereavement services should be made available to families when appropriate. Clinicians should share the burden of making decisions with families and make recommendations based on knowledge about the patient's preferences and values in the context of their clinical condition. For example, "Given what you have told me about your father, and what we know about his medical condition, I recommend...." Knowledge of state laws and institutional policies, common sense, and flexibility are essential when caring for adults with advanced illness who do not have decision-making abilities. Ethics and palliative care consultation can be helpful in difficult cases.[48]

Further Discussion

Case Study

Mr. Smith is 62 years old and has colon cancer. A recent scan reveals progression of disease and new metastases on fourth-line chemotherapeutic agents. A meeting is called to discuss this news and what to do next.

- List six steps to consider using in this family conference to communicate the serious news and establish patient-centered goals of care and a couple of key points for each.

- Mr. Smith and his wife begin by asking you about his prognosis. Given that he has a normal intake but is totally dependent on his wife for his care and completely bed bound, what Palliative Performance Scale (pp. 157-158) category does he fit in?

continued

- Mr. Smith and his wife want to go on a cruise in 6 months. What percentage of patients at his stage of illness will be alive in 6 months?

- What would you tell the patient and his wife about planning this cruise?

The patient and his family want your opinion about his prognosis. You have talked to his oncologist as well as the hospice medical director, and both agree he qualifies for hospice (more likely than not to die in 6 months). You believe that his prognosis is probably shorter than that (2 to 4 months).

- How would you go about telling him his prognosis in a way that preserves hope but also allows him to prepare? Be sure to allow for outliers.

- During the meeting, Mrs. Smith starts to sob loudly, and tears roll from Mr. Smith's eyes. What statement could you make that would

  — acknowledge the emotion

  — legitimize the feelings

  — further explore feelings and reactions

  — empathize

  — explore strengths and coping strategies.

- When patients say that they want everything in response to a conversation about limit setting (eg, DNR/DNI), what might that mean, and how would you approach them as a next step?

Mr. Jones is 78 years old and suffered a large hypertensive intracerebral hemorrhage. Three days after the onset of the stroke, his clinical exams worsen and he now has fixed and dilated pupils but an intact gag reflex, extensor posturing, and spontaneous respirations. After rounding, you plan to meet with his wife and two children to discuss prognosis.

- Describe the steps you would follow to run an optimal family meeting.

- How would you estimate Mr. Jones's prognosis and how would you communicate this to the family?

- Would you expect the family members' prognosis to be different than yours? If so, describe how and why this may be the case.

- What approaches would you use to try and resolve any discrepancies or conflicts that may arise?

References

1. McNutt RA. Shared medical decision making: problems, process, progress. *JAMA.* 2004;292(20):2516-2518.

2. Epstein RM, Peters E. Beyond information: exploring patients' preferences. *JAMA.* 2009;302(2):195-197.

3. Elwyn G, Frosch D, Thomson R, et al. Shared decision making: a model for clinical practice. *J Gen Intern Med.* 2012;27(10):1361-1367.

4. Quill TE. Perspectives on care at the close of life. Initiating end-of-life discussions with seriously ill patients: addressing the "elephant in the room." *JAMA.* 2000;284(19):2502-2507.

5. O'Neill LB, Back AL. What are the key elements to having a conversation about setting goals and communicating serious news? Chapter 43. In: Goldstein NE, Morrison RS, eds. *Evidence-Based Practice of Palliative Medicine: Expert Consult.* New York, NY: Saunders; 2013.

6. Wood GJ, Campbell TC. *Communication and Teamwork. UNIPAC 5.* 4th ed. Glenview, IL: American Academy of Hospice and Palliative Medicine; 2012.

7. Truog RD, Campbell ML, Curtis JR, et al. Recommendations for end-of-life care in the intensive care unit: a consensus statement by the American College of Critical Care Medicine. *Crit Care Med.* 2008;36(3):953-963.

8. Barclay JS, Blackhall LJ, Tulsky JA. Communication strategies and cultural issues in the delivery of bad news. *J Palliat Med.* 2007;10(4):958-977.

9. Quill TE, Arnold RM, Platt F. "I wish things were different": expressing wishes in response to loss, futility, and unrealistic hopes. *Ann Intern Med.* 2001;135(7):551-555.

10. Back AL, Arnold RM, Quill TE. Hope for the best, and prepare for the worst. *Ann Intern Med.* 2003;138(5):439-443.

11. Back AL, Arnold RM. Dealing with conflict in caring for the seriously ill: "it was just out of the question." *JAMA.* 2005;293(11):1374-1381.

12. Buckman R. *How to Break Bad News: A Guide for Health Care Professionals.* Baltimore, MD: The Johns Hopkins University Press; 1992.

13. Quill TE, Arnold R, Back AL. Discussing treatment preferences with patients who want "everything." *Ann Intern Med.* 2009;151(5):345-349.

14. Fisher R, Ury W, Patton B. *Getting to Yes: Negotiating Agreement Without Giving In.* 2nd ed. New York, NY: Penguin Books; 1991.

15. Ahalt C, Walter LC, Yourman L, Eng C, Perez-Stable EJ, Smith AK. "Knowing is better": preferences of diverse older adults for discussing prognosis. *J Gen Intern Med.* 2012;27(5):568-575.

16. Quill TE, Holloway R. Time-limited trials near the end of life. *JAMA.* 2011;306(13):1483-1484.

17. Quinones-Gonzalez S. Bridging the communication gap in hospice and palliative care for Hispanics and Latinos. *Omega (Westport).* 2013;67(1-2):193-200.

18. Casarett DJ, Quill TE. "I'm not ready for hospice": strategies for timely and effective hospice discussions. *Ann Intern Med.* 2007;146(6):443-449.

19. Teno JM, Gozalo PL, Bynum JP, et al. Change in end-of-life care for Medicare beneficiaries: site of death, place of care, and health care transitions in 2000, 2005, and 2009. *JAMA.* 2013;309(5):470-477.

20. National Hospice and Palliative Care Organization. 2013 NHPCO facts and figures: hospice care in america. www.nhpco.org/sites/default/files/public/Statistics_Research/2013_Facts_Figures.pdf. Accessed December 15, 2013.

21. Glare PA, Sinclair CT. Palliative medicine review: prognostication. *J Palliat Med.* 2008;11(1):84-103.

22. Clayton JM, Hancock KM, Butow PN, et al. Clinical practice guidelines for communicating prognosis and end-of-life issues with adults in the advanced stages of a life-limiting illness, and their caregivers. *Med J Aust.* 2007;186(12 Suppl):S77, S79, S83-108.

23. Christakis NA, Lamont EB. Extent and determinants of error in physicians' prognoses in terminally ill patients: prospective cohort study. *West J Med.* 2000;172(5):310-313.

24. Holloway RG, Benesch CG, Burgin WS, Zentner JB. Prognosis and decision making in severe stroke. *JAMA.* 2005;294(6):725-733.

25. Krishnan M, Temel JS, Wright AA, Bernacki R, Selvaggi K, Balboni T. Predicting life expectancy in patients with advanced incurable cancer: a review. *J Support Oncol.* 2013;11(2):68-74.

26. Carroll T, Epstein RM, Gramling R. What is a useful strategy for estimating survival in palliative care settings for persons with advanced cancer? Chapter 41. In: Goldstein NE, Morrison RS, eds. *Evidence-Based Practice of Palliative Medicine.* New York, NY: Elsevier Saunders; 2012.

27. Carroll T, Epstein RM, Gramling R. What is a useful strategy for estimating survival in palliative care settings for persons with advanced non-cancer related illness in palliative care settings? Chapter 42. In: Goldstein NE, Morrison RS, eds. *Evidence-Based Practice of Palliative Medicine.* New York, NY: Elsevier Saunders; 2012.

28. Ripamonti CI, Farina G, Garassino MC. Predictive models in palliative care. *Cancer.* 2009;115(13 Suppl):3128-3134.

29. The STROBE Initiative. Strobe statement: strengthening the reporting of observational studies in epidemiology. www.strobe-statement.org. Accessed August 28, 2013.

30. Victoria Hospice Society. Palliative performance scale. Victoria hospice website. www.victoriahospice.org/health-care-professionals/clinical-tools. Accessed August 28, 2013.

31. Lau F, Maida V, Downing M, Lesperance M, Karlson N, Kuziemsky C. Use of the Palliative Performance Scale (PPS) for end-of-life prognostication in a palliative medicine consultation service. *J Pain Symptom Manage.* 2009;37(6):965-972.

32. Wijdicks EF, Hijdra A, Young GB, Bassetti CL, Wiebe S. Practice parameter: prediction of outcome in comatose survivors after cardiopulmonary resuscitation (an evidence-based review): report of the Quality Standards Subcommittee of the American Academy of Neurology. *Neurology.* 2006;67(2):203-210.

33. Trajkovic-Vidakovic M, de Graeff A, Voest EE, Teunissen SC. Symptoms tell it all: a systematic review of the value of symptom assessment to predict survival in advanced cancer patients. *Crit Rev Oncol Hematol.* 2012;84(1):130-148.

34. Strand K, Flaatten H. Severity scoring in the ICU: a review. *Acta Anaesthesiol Scand.* 2008;52(4):467-478.

35. Simmons BB, Parks SM. Intracerebral hemorrhage for the palliative care provider: what you need to know. *J Palliat Med.* 2008;11(10):1336-1339.

36. Mitchell SL, Kiely DK, Hamel MB, Park PS, Morris JN, Fries BE. Estimating prognosis for nursing home residents with advanced dementia. *JAMA.* 2004;291(22):2734-2740.

37. Lee M, Chodosh J. Dementia and life expectancy: what do we know? *J Am Med Dir Assoc.* 2009;10(7):466-471.

38. Lamont EB, Christakis NA. Complexities in prognostication in advanced cancer: "to help them live their lives the way they want to." *JAMA.* 2003;290(1):98-104.

39. Abrahm JL, Banffy MB, Harris MB. Spinal cord compression in patients with advanced metastatic cancer: "all I care about is walking and living my life." *JAMA.* 2008;299(8):937-946.

40. Victoria Palliative Research Network. Prognostat. Palliative Performance Scale. https://htg.his.uvic.ca/tools/PrognosticTools/PalliativePerformanceScale/index.php. Accessed August 29, 2013.

41. ePrognosis. Estimating prognosis for elders. http://eprognosis.ucsf.edu. Accessed August 29, 2013.

42. Levy WC, Mozaffarian D, Linker DT. Seattle Heart Failure Model. University of Washington website. http://depts.washington.edu/shfm. Accessed August 29, 2013.

43. Perel P, Arango M, Clayton T, et al. Predicting outcome after traumatic brain injury: practical prognostic models based on large cohort of international patients. *BMJ*. 2008;336(7641):425-429.

44. Cote T, Kinzbrunner B, eds. *The Hospice Medical Director Manual*. 2nd ed. Glenview, IL: American Academy of Hospice and Palliative Medicine; 2012.

45. Ngo-Metzger Q, August KJ, Srinivasan M, Liao S, Meyskens FL, Jr. End-of-life care: guidelines for patient-centered communication. *Am Fam Physician*. 2008;77(2):167-174.

46. Berger JT, DeRenzo EG, Schwartz J. Surrogate decision making: reconciling ethical theory and clinical practice. *Ann Intern Med*. 2008;149(1):48-53.

47. Hudson P, Quinn K, O'Hanlon B, Aranda S. Family meetings in palliative care: multidisciplinary clinical practice guidelines. *BMC Palliat Care*. 2008;7:12.

48. Rincon F, Lee K. Ethical considerations in consenting critically ill patients for bedside clinical care and research. *J Intensive Care Med*. 2013.

49. Shalowitz DI, Garrett-Mayer E, Wendler D. The accuracy of surrogate decision makers: a systematic review. *Arch Intern Med*. 2006;166(5):493-497.

50. Boyd EA, Lo B, Evans LR, et al. "It's not just what the doctor tells me": factors that influence surrogate decision-makers' perceptions of prognosis. *Crit Care Med*. 2010;38(5):1270-1275.

51. Zier LS, Sottile PD, Hong SY, Weissfield LA, White DB. Surrogate decision makers' interpretation of prognostic information: a mixed-methods study. *Ann Intern Med*. 2012;156(5):360-366.

52. Wendler D, Rid A. Systematic review: the effect on surrogates of making treatment decisions for others. *Ann Intern Med*. 2011;154(5):336-346.

EIGHT

Last-Resort Options

8A | Proportionate Palliative Sedation

Proportionate palliative sedation, potentially to the level of unconsciousness, is the use of progressively higher levels of sedation to help relieve otherwise intractable and distressing physical symptoms at the very end of a patient's life.[1-5] The purpose of the sedation is to relieve otherwise uncontrollable suffering, not to intentionally end a patient's life or hasten a patient's death. Sedation is therefore consistent with standard palliative care practice. Because these patients are imminently dying (usually within 2 weeks), withholding or withdrawing other life-sustaining therapies as part of the process, such as mechanical ventilators or artificial hydration and nutrition, should be strongly considered but treated as a separate clinical decision.

This intervention should be applied when the goal of treatment is to cause sedation as the means of alleviating otherwise intractable and distressing physical symptoms. (See Chapter 5 for addressing seemingly intractable psychological, spiritual, and existential suffering.) Examples of conditions when proportionate palliative sedation might be initiated include agitated terminal delirium, unrelenting nausea and vomiting, intractable pain, and unrelenting dyspnea in actively dying patients who do not respond to the usual palliative treatments. The aim of treatment is to achieve the lowest level of sedation that adequately relieves the patient's symptoms. Other potential symptom-relieving measures should be continued as sedation is added. Proportionate palliative sedation should be distinguished from *ordinary sedation* (the use of sedatives to assist with sleep or to treat anxiety when consciousness and alertness is preserved) and *palliative sedation to unconsciousness* (a more controversial practice in which unconsciousness is the intended end point needed to relieve otherwise intolerable suffering).[1] Although unconsciousness may eventually be the outcome of proportionate palliative sedation, it is not the intended aim nor is it inevitable. If lesser levels of sedation are sufficient to relieve the patient's suffering, then the dosage of sedating medication is not increased further with this practice. Relieving the patient's suffering using the minimum level of sedation necessary is the essence of proportionate palliative sedation. **If rapid sedation to unconsciousness is felt to be the best approach because of the patient's unique clinical circumstances, then it is critical to have experts in palliative care and ethics involved before initiation to ensure all other approaches have been fully considered and the circumstances warrant the intervention.**

Terminally ill patients receiving proportionate palliative sedation should have do-not-resuscitate (DNR) and do-not-intubate (DNI) orders before the treatment is initiated. Patients with capacity should provide verbal or written consent prior to initiating the process because capacity usually will be compromised once it is started. If the patient lacks capacity from the start, the decision to initiate proportionate palliative sedation would be made by the patient's surrogate decision maker(s) using substituted judgment in a manner consistent with decisions to withhold or withdraw potentially life-prolonging treatments. The healthcare team should document all elements of the clinical decision in the medical record, including the exact nature of the intractable suffering, the alternative treatments that have been tried, the consultations that have been obtained, and the consent or decision-making process involving the patient (if the patient still has capacity), family, or close friends.

Formal *palliative care consultation*, if available, is strongly recommended before proportionate palliative sedation is initiated for guidance in the process and to ensure that all other palliative measures have been fully considered. If there is uncertainty about the adequacy of pain management, a pain service consultation also is recommended. If there is uncertainty about the appropriateness of the practice with a given patient, especially if palliative sedation to unconsciousness is being considered, an ethics consultation is recommended. Full involvement of the patient's family is encouraged at each step unless contrary to the patient's wishes. If artificial nutrition and hydration are simultaneously stopped, death usually occurs within days to weeks.

Guidelines for Initiating Proportionate Palliative Sedation

Following a decision by the patient or surrogate and the patient's attending physician, and after appropriate consultation, palliative sedation orders are written according to **Table 8.1**. The healthcare team should adhere to the following guidelines:

1. If hospitalized, the patient should be transferred to a private room and if at home, hospice inpatient admission should be considered. Family should be allowed unlimited visiting unless it is contrary to the patient's wishes.
2. The decision-making process and plan should be discussed with the nursing staff on the patient care unit to ensure they understand what is being ordered and why.
3. The healthcare team should obtain and document a baseline assessment, including refractory symptoms (ie, delirium, shortness of breath, pain), sedation or agitation level (see **Table 8.2**), other vital signs, any additional signs or symptoms of suffering, and any treatments that had been previously tried and found ineffective.
4. The healthcare team should continue currently effective symptom-relieving measures alongside the sedation.

The healthcare team should administer sedating medication per the following order:

1. Initiate infusion. A medical provider should be present at initiation of infusion and be available until the patient exhibits signs of refractory-symptom stabilization.
2. Monitor the levels of sedation or agitation. The lowest level of sedation (see Sedation Agitation Scale in Table 8.2) needed to control the patient's refractory symptoms should be the goal.
3. If symptoms are unrelieved at agreed-upon time intervals (the range may be minutes to hours to days, depending on the severity of the symptoms being treated), give an additional bolus and increase the sedative infusion rate in 20% to 30% increments.

Once adequate symptom relief is achieved, maintain the patient on the infusion rate that achieved the relief. Assess and document the following at least every 2 hours:

- level of symptom relief
- level of sedation
- patient, family, or significant other's coping.

Adjust the infusion upward if uncomfortable symptoms recur. Family members and significant others should be allowed to remain with the patient and participate in care, if desired, to the fullest extent possible.

Ensure family support during the process of proportionate palliative sedation to emphasize the ongoing intent of the sedation, inform the family members of changes during the dying process, and attend to the emotional needs and anticipatory grief of the family.[6]

Table 8.1 Medications for Palliative Sedation*

MEDICATION	DOSAGE	COMMENT
Midazolam	Bolus: 0.5 mg-2.5 mg IV push over 2 minutes	Medication most often used for palliative sedation
	Maintenance: 0.02 mg-0.2 mg/kg/hour	
	Routes: IV or SC	
Lorazepam	Bolus: 1 mg-4 mg every 4 to 6 hours PO or dissolved buccally, or 0.5 mg-2 mg IV bolus	
	Maintenance: 0.01 mg-0.1 mg/kg/hour	
	Routes: PO, SC, IV, buccal	
Phenobarbitol	Bolus: 200 mg slow IV injection repeated every 10 to 15 minutes until comfortable	Long-acting
	Maintenance: 60 mg-180 mg twice a day; plus 60 mg every hour prn	
	Routes: IV or SC (may also be compounded as a rectal suppository)	

IV, intravenous; PO, oral; SC, subcutaneous.
Opioids used to treat pain or dyspnea should be continued in this process.

Table 8.2 Sedation Agitation Scale

SCORE	LEVEL OF SEDATION	SIGNS AND SYMPTOMS
7	Dangerous agitation	Pulling at endotracheal tube, trying to remove catheters, climbing over bedrails, striking at staff, thrashing side to side
6	Very agitated	Does not calm despite frequent verbal reminders of limits, requires physical restraints, bites endotracheal tube
5	Agitated	Anxious or mildly agitated, makes attempts to sit up, calms down with verbal instructions
4	Calm and cooperative	Calm, awakens easily, follows commands
3	Sedated	Difficult to arouse, awakens to verbal stimuli or gentle shaking but drifts off again, follows simple commands
2	Very sedated	Arouses to physical stimuli but does not communicate or follow commands, may move spontaneously
1	Unarousable	Minimal or no response to noxious stimuli, does not communicate or follow commands

8B | Ventilator Withdrawal

Palliative care teams often are asked to assist with ventilator withdrawal when it has been decided that mechanical ventilation is no longer consistent with a patient's goals of care. Such decisions are never easy for family members or medical practitioners, and palliative care providers can help both by supporting all those involved and by providing recommendations for a comfortable transition for the patient.[7,8]

Preparations immediately before ventilator withdrawal include the following:

- Ensure there is a clear consensus among the patient, family, other surrogates, and clinicians that withdrawal is indicated by the patient's clinical condition and personal values (if the patient cannot express his or her wishes at the current time, by what is known about the patient's values).

- Clearly document the discussions with the patient, family/surrogates, and healthcare providers, including the consensus about the withdrawal decision. Ask about any spiritual or religious activities that may be relevant and encourage the family to make arrangements for any special rituals that may be important to them.
- Set a tentative time for the withdrawal with the family and staff that ensures time for key family members to be present should they choose to be, and also allows adequate time for saying good-bye in case the patient dies quickly. This also ensures sufficient staffing and presence of knowledgeable medical personnel.
- Prepare the family for what to expect, including the potential for restlessness, noisy breathing, the possibility that after extubation the patient may not breathe on his or her own, and an estimate of how long the patient will live (with exceptions in both directions).
- Maintain intravenous access, but turn off all monitors and alarms and discontinue blood pressure medications, paralytic medication, and all medical treatments not immediately necessary for comfort. Continue all treatments that are palliative in intent (opioids, anxiolytics, anticholinergics). If the patient has an implanted defibrillator, it should be deactivated.
- Give family members the option of staying in the room for the extubation or stepping out briefly while the extubation and immediate comfort are attended to.
- Clear a space for the family at the bedside and, if the family has stepped out of the room, invite them back in at the earliest opportunity to touch and talk to the patient, if they desire.

Two methods of ventilator withdrawal—immediate extubation and terminal weaning—have been described. Either method may be appropriate depending on the clinical circumstances, clinician's personal experience and comfort, and patient and family preferences. Immediate extubation is generally the preferred approach. Terminal weaning may be preferred, however, when the volume of secretions is high and the airway is likely to be compromised. Terminal weaning may be carried out over a period of 30 to 60 minutes and involves decreasing the ventilator rate and positive end-expiratory pressure while the endo-tracheal tube (ETT) is left in place. A T-piece can be attached to the ETT if the patient continues to breathe. More details regarding these two methods of ventilator withdrawal are available online at the EPERC website, www.eperc.mcw.edu.[7,9]

An experienced physician and nurse should be present at the time that ventilator withdrawal is initiated to ensure adequate symptom control. Before withdrawing the ventilator, be sure the patient is comfortable and monitor for any signs of respiratory distress. Adjust opioids upward if respiratory distress is present and adjust benzodiazepines or other sedating medications if agitation or restlessness is present. Opioids and benzodiazepines are the primary medications used to provide comfort in this setting, typically in dosages that cause sedation. There is no medical, ethical, or legal justification for withholding sedating medication in this setting, when death following ventilator withdrawal is expected, out of fear of hastening death (see section 8A on proportionate palliative sedation). The amount of sedating medication required will depend on the patient's level of consciousness; the degree of agitation, restlessness, and dyspnea present; and prior use of similar medications. Patients who are conscious may request sedation to the level of unconsciousness before the withdrawal. In these circumstances, rapid and full sedation should be the goal, and a palliative care consult should be obtained (see section 8A). Use of general anesthesia for this purpose remains ethically controversial but has been discussed in the critical care literature.[10,11]

The following are general guidelines for ventilator withdrawal in adults.

- For patients who have not been on opioids or benzodiazepines, shortly before withdrawal give a 2 mg to 10 mg IV bolus of morphine or equivalent, followed by an infusion of 1 mg to 5 mg IV per hour, as well as a 1 mg to 2 mg IV bolus of midazolam or lorazepam followed by an infusion of 1 mg to 2 mg IV per hour.

- If the patient is already on continuous opioids or anxiolytics, give a bolus of two times the current hourly rate, then increase the hourly infusion rate by 30%.
- Rapidly titrate these medications upward as needed to minimize shortness of breath, restlessness, and anxiety and to achieve an adequate level of comfort.
- If distress ensues after ventilator withdrawal, aggressive and immediate symptom control is imperative. Use morphine, 5 mg to 10 mg IV every 10 minutes (or 10% of the patient's total daily infusion rate) and midazolam, 2 mg to 4 mg IV every 10 minutes as needed. Adjust both infusion rates upward in 30% increments until distress is relieved.
- Specific dosages are less important than achieving symptom relief. A general goal is to keep the respiratory rate under 30 (and ideally under 20) and to eliminate grimacing and agitation.

If it appears that the patient has only a short time to live, and the resources are available, it is advisable to keep the patient in the intensive care unit until he or she dies to ensure comfort. However, if the patient continues to breathe on his or her own and appears to have a longer time to live, transfer to a medical floor or a palliative care unit may be appropriate. In this case, communication with the nursing staff is paramount to ensure that appropriate palliative measures are provided to the patient. Titration orders for continuous infusions should be made clear to the nursing staff to ensure immediate adjustments can be made if the patient develops worsening symptoms. Continue to support family members and encourage them to voice any questions or concerns they may have. After death occurs, encourage the family to spend as much time at the bedside as they desire and provide bereavement and grief support.

8C | Evaluating Suicide Risk in Terminal Illness

The prevalence of suicidal ideation and suicide attempts among the terminally ill population has not been widely studied, but evidence suggests vulnerability to suicide increases when patients have advanced illness with a poor prognosis and suffer from depression, anxiety, or hopelessness.[12,13] Clinicians caring for seriously ill patients need to have a high index of suspicion for subtle or direct expression of suicidal ideation and an awareness of risk factors as outlined in **Table 8.3**. Clinicians also need to have a clear strategy for evaluating and responding to requests for hastened death in seriously ill patients.

Table 8.3 Risk Factors for Suicide in Patients with Advanced Disease

RELATED TO DISEASE
Uncontrolled pain

Advanced disease and poor prognosis

Pharyngeal, lung, gastrointestinal, urogenital, or breast cancer

Advanced HIV disease

Exhaustion and fatigue

RELATED TO MENTAL STATUS
Depression and hopelessness

Delirium and disinhibition

Psychotic features (eg, hallucinations and delusions)

Loss of control and impulsiveness

Irrational thinking

Persistent suicidal ideation and lethal plans

Loss of perceived functioning

Severe existential distress

RELATED TO PERSONAL AND FAMILY HISTORY
Preexisting psychiatric disease (eg, major depression, anxiety disorders)

Substance abuse (eg, alcohol)

Recent loss (eg, spouse or friends)

Lack of social supports

Older age, male sex

Prior suicide attempts and family history of suicide

Loss of self-identified role (eg, parent, employer, worker)

Fears of being a burden

8D | Evaluating Requests for Hastened Death in Terminal Illness[14]*

It is not uncommon for a patient to request a healthcare professional's help in hastening death. The motivation for this request generally stems from a combination of relentless physical symptoms, progressive debility, loss of sense of self, loss of control, fear of the future, and fear of being a burden on others. It can also be a cry for help in the setting of an acute and sudden illness or devastating diagnosis. Some physicians are frightened by these requests, feeling that they are being asked to cross unacceptable professional boundaries. Others may be tempted to quickly accede, imagining that they would want the same thing if they were in the patient's shoes. But requests for a hastened death may provide an introduction into a patient's experience of suffering and may lead to opportunities for more effective treatment if fully evaluated.[14,15,16] In general, the clinician should carefully clarify, explore, evaluate, and intensify treatment and support to ensure a full understanding of the request and that all alternatives have been considered. This section provides guidance on how to evaluate and initially respond to a patient who raises the topic of a hastened death. The next section will explore how to respond when the request for a hastened death persists after a full evaluation, and how to search for remedies to the patient's underlying problems.

- Clarify exactly what is being asked before responding. Is the patient simply having thoughts or worries about dying (very common)? Is he or she contemplating the possibility of a hastened death in the future if his or her suffering becomes overwhelming? Is he or she exploring a wish to end his or her life right now?[17,18]

- Support the patient and family. Reinforce your commitment to try to find a solution for the patient's problem and assure the patient that you will continue to care for him or her no matter what happens. This means searching in earnest with the patient and family to find a mutually acceptable way to approach the patient's dilemma.[19] Attend

---

*From Quill TE, Arnold R. Evaluating requests for hastened death. Fast Facts and Concepts #156. Milwaukee, WI: End of Life/Palliative Education Resource Center; 2009. Adapted with permission.

to your own support by discussing the patient's request with trusted colleagues or with your interdisciplinary team.

- Evaluate the patient's decision-making capacity. Is the patient seeing his or her medical condition clearly? Is the request proportionate to the level of unrelieved suffering? Are there dominating aspects of anhedonia, worthlessness, and guilt, or is the capacity for pleasure and joy preserved in some small way? Is this request consistent with the patient's past values? Request help from an experienced psychiatrist or psychologist if you are unsure.[15,20]

- Explore the many potential dimensions that may contribute to the patient's unbearable suffering to be sure you (and the patient) fully understand its underlying cause(s). It may be an unrelenting physical symptom, feelings of depression, a family or spiritual crisis, or perhaps a combination of many factors.

- Respond to the associated emotions, which may be strong and conflicted. Try to imagine what the patient is going through. Distinguish your own feelings and reactions from those of the patient.[21]

- Intensify treatment of any potentially reversible elements of the patient's suffering. Depending on the patient's circumstances, offer to increase treatment of pain or other physical symptoms, and consider pharmacological and interpersonal treatment of depression (see section 5B [p. 100]). Help the patient find an appropriate and acceptable spiritual counselor. Be creative, and brainstorm potential solutions with your interdisciplinary team.

- Respond directly to the request for hastened death only after this multidimensional evaluation has been completed. If the patient has full decision-making capacity and all alternative approaches to the patient's unbearable suffering have been fully considered, then re-explore exactly what is being requested and look for mutually acceptable ways to potentially respond.[22,23] Note that many patients may be looking for the potential of an escape they will never use, but a smaller number will be looking for a way to hasten death in the present.

8E | Responding to Persistent Requests for Hastened Death[24]‡

With good symptom management and psychological and spiritual support, most patients do not persist in their request for a hastened death. This section focuses on ways to respond to patients who continue to want a hastened death despite every effort to find appropriate palliative care alternatives.[22,23] This section applies only to patients with full decision-making capacity. It does not address requests for a hastened death from surrogate decision makers, which should be fully explored and understood, but then responded to with further intensification of accepted palliative treatments. Every effort should be made to evaluate and understand the request and then jointly search for other acceptable ways of responding.

Reflect on your personal feelings about the request and discuss with other professionals. These cases are emotionally and ethically difficult. Brainstorm options with other members of the care team including physician colleagues, nurses, psychologists, chaplains, and others. Allow trusted colleagues to support your emotional reactions.

Seek out consultation or a second opinion. Make sure you understand the medical, legal, and ethical issues involved in responding to a particular request for hastened death. Palliative care and ethics consultations can be invaluable. Independent second opinions may be helpful in clarifying the prognosis and ensuring that all potentially effective therapeutic alternatives have been considered.

Learn the possibilities for resolving the patient's request. The possibilities are listed below from least to most ethically controversial. Considering these possibilities assumes that aggressive measures to control physical, psychological, and spiritual suffering have been exhausted.

- *Withdrawal of life-sustaining treatments.* Although most clinicians consider stopping invasive treatments (eg, ventilators, implanted defibrillators, feeding tubes) under these circumstances, simpler therapies such as a pacemaker, insulin, antibiotics, or steroids might

‡*Adapted with permission from Quill T, Arnold R. Responding to a request for hastened death. Fast Facts and Concepts #159. Fast Facts and Concepts. Milwaukee, WI: End of Life/Palliative Education Resource Center; 2009.*

also be voluntarily discontinued if they are prolonging life against the patient's wishes. (There is widespread legal and ethical consensus about the permissibility of this response based on a patient's right to bodily integrity.)[7-9]

- *Proportionate palliative sedation, potentially to the level of unconsciousness.* This practice is used for relief of severe intractable physical symptoms in the imminently dying patient (see section 8A). Consciousness is preserved to the extent possible, but sometimes the level of suffering is so severe that its relief requires consciousness to be significantly diminished. The intent of sedation is to relieve intolerable suffering, but the only remaining means to do so is by a reduction in patient consciousness. If artificial hydration and feeding are simultaneously stopped, death will usually occur within 1 to 2 weeks.[1]

- *Voluntary cessation of oral intake.* Patients may choose to stop eating and drinking as a means to hasten the dying process. Completely stopping oral food and liquids will typically result in death within 2 weeks. (Small amounts of food and water can extend this time frame substantially.)

- *Physician-assisted death* (also called physician-assisted suicide). A physician provides the means (eg, usually a potentially lethal prescription for barbiturates) for a patient to voluntarily end his or her life. The patient decides if and when the medicine is actually used, and the patient is responsible for and must be capable of taking the medicine him- or herself. As of 2013, physician-assisted death is illegal in the United States except in Oregon, Washington, Montana, and Vermont.

Decision-making process. Have a detailed conversation regarding the risks and benefits of the different possibilities that fit the patient's clinical circumstances and that the patient, family, and you find ethically acceptable. Be as specific as possible and clearly document your thought process. Your intent must always be to relieve otherwise intolerable suffering. Be sure everyone understands that all standard palliative care alternatives have been at least considered if not tried. Informed consent must be obtained from the patient or surrogate decision maker acting on his or her behalf.

Balance integrity and nonabandonment.[19] It is not always possible to find common ground between the patient and physician. When asked to support a particular act, a physician needs to be as specific as possible about what he or she can and cannot do and why. Although physicians should not violate personal principles to respond to a request they find unacceptable, they should search in earnest with the patient and family for alternative options that might be mutually acceptable. Typically, this approach will allow the physician to maintain integrity while not abandoning the patient, even if agreement about the particular act being requested is not possible.

Further Discussion

1. What are the differences between usual indications for proportionate palliative sedation and palliative sedation to unconsciousness?

2. A patient with advanced lung cancer had been DNR and DNI on home hospice when he became acutely short of breath, panicked, and came to the emergency department where he was intubated. He is now sedated and on a ventilator. You discuss the situation with his primary doctor and his oncologist, and then meet with the family. All agree that he never wanted this and would want to be allowed to die peacefully off machines. He currently is on a lorazepam drip at 0.5 mg/hr and hydromorphone drip at 2 mg/hr, and he appears comfortable. Before taking him off the ventilator, what should you do with his drips, and how rapidly should you be ready to provide prn medications?

3. Name two risk factors for mental-illness-related suicide in each of the following categories:
   - disease types
   - mental status factors
   - personal and family history.

4. Your patient with advanced congestive heart failure has been in the hospital for 2 weeks receiving maximal medical treatment including intravenous inotropic therapy. He tells the nurses he wants to "get it over with." You are asked to evaluate him. What should be your initial response?

5. What are potentially confounding factors that might underlie this statement?

6. Who else should you discuss this statement with?

7. You discuss this patient with both the heart failure and the palliative care teams. There is agreement that (a) medical treatment has been maximized, (b) prognosis is very poor, (c) clinical depression is not distorting his judgment, and (d) his dyspnea and depression are being maximally managed. The patient is frightened about waiting for the next severe shortness of breath exacerbation to arise before he dies and wants to know if he has any other options.

   • Which of the last-resort options are potentially available to this patient?

   • Which option(s) would best address his situation?

   • Of these potential options, are there any you could not support?

References

1. Quill TE, Lo B, Brock DW, Meisel A. Last-resort options for palliative sedation. *Ann Intern Med*. 2009;151(6):421-424.

2. Sykes N, Thorns A. Sedative use in the last week of life and the implications for end-of-life decision making. *Arch Intern Med*. 2003;163(3):341-344.

3. Quill TE, Byock IR. Responding to intractable terminal suffering: the role of terminal sedation and voluntary refusal of food and fluids. ACP-ASIM End-of-Life Care Consensus Panel. American College of Physicians-

American Society of Internal Medicine. *Ann Intern Med.* 2000;132(5): 408-414.

4. Swart SJ, van der Heide A, van Zuylen L, et al. Considerations of physicians about the depth of palliative sedation at the end of life. *CMAJ.* 2012;184(7):E360-366.

5. Maltoni M, Scarpi E, Rosati M, et al. Palliative sedation in end-of-life care and survival: a systematic review. *J Clin Oncol.* 2012;30(12):1378-1383.

6. Bruinsma SM, Rietjens JA, Seymour JE, Anquinet L, van der Heide A. The experiences of relatives with the practice of palliative sedation: a systematic review. *J Pain Symptom Manage.* 2012;44(3):431-445.

7. von Gunten C, Weissman DE. Symptom control for ventilator withdrawal in the dying patient. *Fast Facts and Concepts #34.* Milwaukee, WI: End of Life/Palliative Education Resource Center; 2009. www.mcw.edu/FileLibrary/User/jrehm/fastfactpdfs/Concept034.pdf. Accessed October 12, 2013.

8. von Gunten C, Weissman DE. Information for patients and families about ventilator withdrawal. *Fast Facts and Concepts #35.* Milwaukee, WI: End of Life/Palliative Education Resource Center; 2009. www.mcw.edu/FileLibrary/User/jrehm/fastfactpdfs/Concept035.pdf. Accessed October 12, 2013.

9. von Gunten C, Weissman DE. Ventilator withdrawal protocol. *Fast Facts and Concepts #33.* Milwaukee, WI: End of Life/Palliative Education Resource Center; 2009. www.mcw.edu/FileLibrary/User/jrehm/fastfactpdfs/Concept033.pdf. Accessed October 12, 2013.

10. Billings JA. Humane terminal extubation reconsidered: the role for preemptive analgesia and sedation. *Crit Care Med.* 2012;40(2):625-630.

11. Truog RD, Brock DW, White DB. Should patients receive general anesthesia prior to extubation at the end of life? *Crit Care Med.* 2012;40(2):631-633.

12. Breitbart W, Rosenfeld B, Pessin H, et al. Depression, hopelessness, and desire for hastened death in terminally ill patients with cancer. *JAMA.* 2000;284(22):2907-2911.

13. Chochinov HM, Wilson KG, Enns M, et al. Desire for death in the terminally ill. *Am J Psychiatry.* 1995;152(8):1185-1191.

14. Quill TE, Arnold R. Evaluating requests for hastened death. *Fast Facts and Concepts #156.* Milwaukee, WI: End of Life/Palliative Education Resource

Center; 2009. www.eperc.mcw.edu/EPERC/FastFactsIndex/ff_156.htm. Accessed December 13, 2013.

15. Ganzini L, Goy ER, Dobscha SK. Prevalence of depression and anxiety in patients requesting physicians' aid in dying: cross sectional survey. *BMJ.* 2008;337:a1682.

16. Ganzini L, Goy ER, Dobscha SK. Oregonians' reasons for requesting physician aid in dying. *Arch Intern Med.* 2009;169(5):489-492.

17. Quill TE. Doctor, I want to die. Will you help me? *JAMA.* 1993;270(7):870-873.

18. Block SD, Billings JA. Patient requests to hasten death. Evaluation and management in terminal care. *Arch Intern Med.* 1994;154(18):2039-2047.

19. Quill TE, Cassel CK. Nonabandonment: a central obligation for physicians. *Ann Intern Med.* 1995;122(5):368-374.

20. Block SD. Assessing and managing depression in the terminally ill patient. ACP-ASIM End-of-Life Care Consensus Panel. American College of Physicians—American Society of Internal Medicine. *Ann Intern Med.* 2000;132(3):209-218.

21. Meier DE, Back AL, Morrison RS. The inner life of physicians and care of the seriously ill. *JAMA.* 2001;286(23):3007-3014.

22. Quill TE, Lo B, Brock DW. Palliative options of last resort: a comparison of voluntarily stopping eating and drinking, terminal sedation, physician-assisted suicide, and voluntary active euthanasia. *JAMA.* 1997;278(23):2099-2104.

23. Quill TE, Lee BC, Nunn S. Palliative treatments of last resort: choosing the least harmful alternative. University of Pennsylvania Center for Bioethics Assisted Suicide Consensus Panel. *Ann Intern Med.* 2000;132(6):488-493.

24. Quill TE, Arnold R. Responding to a request for hastened death. *Fast Facts and Concepts #159.* Milwaukee, WI: End of Life/Palliative Education Resource Center; 2009. www.eperc.mcw.edu/EPERC/FastFactsIndex/ff_159.htm. Accessed October 10, 2013.

NINE

Care During the Last Hours of Life

9A | What to Prepare For

How do you know if a patient is actively dying? Physicians' prognoses tend to be inaccurate for most terminal patients and, if anything, physicians err by being overly optimistic.[1] There are, however, some clinical signs that indicate death is imminent.[2] Actively dying patients usually are bedbound, extremely weak, barely communicative, and rarely able to swallow sufficient amounts of fluid. Changes in circulation (causing dusky or cyanotic hands and feet) and breathing (including long periods of apnea and very shallow breaths) and an inability to handle the mucous in the throat, often causing the patient to gurgle on expiration ("death rattle"), are common.

Although most health professionals have seen dying patients, the general public rarely witnesses the process of dying. The popular media have created dramatizations and sometimes false expectations of the dying experience. Those who provide care to the actively dying have the opportunity to help patients and their families prepare for the final hours of life. If managed poorly, both the patient and family may experience unnecessary suffering, and family distress may continue long after the patient's death.[3] When the last hours are managed well, however, most patients are comforted at the time of their death, and their families and friends experience a positive first step in their bereavement. Effective teamwork is essential to obtaining these results.

Preparation for the dying experience often should occur from the beginning of palliative care involvement. As the last days and hours of life approach, the family and other caregivers may need greater emotional support and more detailed information about what they might witness during the dying experience. Most patients in the final stages of terminal illness benefit from the 24-hour presence of caregivers—family, professionals, or both. If family members are caring for the patient at home with hospice support, two family members ideally should be present to provide mutual support to one another as well as to the patient. This is a time when an experienced hospice and palliative care team can be particularly helpful. If members of the team recognize that a patient is actively dying, they should communicate this to the patient, relatives, and other caregivers in a calm, reassuring way.[2] This information allows for adequate preparation by those who will witness the last hours of life and also allows the care team to remain alert for new problems and adapt the care plan quickly to address concerns.

It is crucial to have medications and equipment readily available in anticipation of terminal symptoms, including pain, dyspnea, anxiety, restlessness, or secretions.[4,5]

Families may need to have the following medications in the home[4]:

- **For pain and dyspnea:** concentrated opioid (eg, morphine liquid concentrate 20 mg/mL)
- **For anxiety and agitation:** concentrated benzodiazepine (eg, lorazepam liquid 2 mg/mL)
- **For nausea or restlessness:** haloperidol or lorazepam liquid, crushed tablets, or prochlorperazine suppository
- **For secretions:** anticholinergic (eg, glycopyrrolate, hyoscyamine, or atropine to give sublingually or scopolamine patches).

In the institutional setting, appropriate care pathways and medication orders need to be in place to ensure effective symptom management, including adequate medications to address common symptoms (similar to those listed above); documentation of the patient's advance directives, including do-not-resuscitate (DNR) status; and other orders to maximize the patient's comfort and minimize discomfort (eg, discontinuing monitors, vital signs, and all treatments not geared toward immediate comfort). In addition, the last hours of care in institutions (eg, nursing home, hospital) frequently provide a significant opportunity for education and support for staff members who, in addition to family members, also may be struggling with the dying experience. Never assume that dying is a normal or common part of a healthcare professional's experience.

In preparing families and professional caregivers for the visible changes that will occur as death approaches, it is helpful to discuss physiologic changes that commonly occur in the last hours to days of life.[3]

Weakness and Fatigue

The patient will gradually lose mobility. Movements in bed may become difficult, joints may become pained and stiff, and the potential for developing pressure ulcers will increase. To minimize the risk of pressure ulcer formation, the patient can be gently turned or repositioned regularly. Pillows and blankets can be used to elevate the back, head, or extremities. It is not unusual for patients with significant edema to develop swelling in the extremities or face; often this can be reduced simply by repositioning or elevating against gravity. Turning and repositioning can be uncomfortable for some patients, so it may be appropriate to premedicate such patients with opioid analgesics before repositioning them. As the patient approaches death, the need for turning must be considered in the context of causing potential discomfort and the patient's overall prognosis.

Decreased Food and Fluid Intake

Although decreased oral intake of food and fluids can occur early in terminal illness and result in progressive weight loss, patients and families need to be educated that loss of appetite and development of dehydration are nearly universal prior to death. Many caregivers may be worried that the patient will starve to death or die from dehydration. Families need to be educated that forcing food and fluids actually may lead to discomfort for the patient. Clinicians can help families understand that loss of appetite is normal at this stage of illness and teach them that most patients are not hungry, that food may not be appealing or may be nauseating, and that teeth clenching may be the only way for a nonverbal patient to express desires.

Dehydration also occurs naturally as part of dying and does not need to be associated with thirst or discomfort. As patients develop swallowing difficulties, oral fluid intake can lead to aspiration, choking, and further discomfort. Parenteral fluids can worsen edema, ascites, and pulmonary congestion and in most cases do not contribute to the patient's comfort or longevity.[6] To support the patient's comfort, try to sustain the moisture and hygiene of the mouth, nose, and eyes. Several strategies have been recommended to accomplish this goal:

- Moisten and clean the mouth with a swab as needed using a baking soda solution (1 teaspoon salt, 1 teaspoon baking soda, 1 quart tepid water), plain water, or an artificial saliva preparation. Avoid commercial mouthwashes, which often contain alcohol and can be irritating.
- Treat oral candidiasis (thrush) with topical nystatin suspension or systemic fluconazole (if the patient is able to swallow).
- Frequently coat the lips and anterior nasal mucosa with a thin layer of petroleum jelly. Avoid swabs containing lemon and glycerin because these can be irritating, particularly on open sores. If oxygen is being delivered by nasal cannula, consider humidification to prevent the nasal mucosa from drying.
- If the eyelids are not closed, moisten the conjunctiva with an ophthalmic lubricating gel, artificial tears, or a normal saline solution every 30 minutes to 4 hours.

Decreased Ability to Swallow and Cough

In addition to the loss of the ability to take food and fluids, the process of dying also impairs the cough/gag reflex and the ability to clear secretions and protect the airway from aspiration. The pooling of saliva in the posterior oropharynx and the retention of secretions in the tracheobronchial tree can lead to noisy respirations, including gurgling, crackling, and rattling ("death rattle"). To caregivers, this can be quite disturbing and sound as if the patient is choking. Simple measures such as repositioning the patient can result in postural drainage and effectively relieve some symptoms. Please refer to Table 3.3 for detailed recommendations for the management of respiratory symptoms. Oropharyngeal or nasopharyngeal suctioning generally is not indicated because it can cause considerable discomfort to the patient. In most cases, the secretions are located deeper in the respiratory tract and are not accessible for suctioning. Copious secretions can be reduced with the use of anticholinergic medications.[7] Some treatment options include

- glycopyrrolate, 1 mg to 2 mg orally (PO) two or three times a day (although oral absorption can be unpredictable) or 0.2 mg to 0.4 mg intravenously or subcutaneously (SC) every 4 to 8 hours[8]
- hyoscyamine, 0.125 mg orally disintegrating tablets, 1 or 2 tabs PO (or sublingually [SL]), or 0.125 mg/mL oral solution, 1 mL to 2 mL every 4 hours
  - Both glycopyrrolate and hyoscyamine may be less likely to exacerbate confusion from their anticholinergic effects because neither drug crosses the blood-brain barrier.
- atropine, 1% ophthalmic drops, 1 or 2 drops every 1 to 2 hours as needed (prn)
- scopolamine, 1 to 3 patches transdermally (TD) every 3 days, or 0.4 mg SC every 4 to 6 hours prn.

Reduced Circulation and Renal Function

Dehydration and reduced cardiac output result in reduced peripheral perfusion, causing extremities to appear cyanotic and feel cool to the touch. Patients may develop tachycardia and hypotension. Decreased renal perfusion eventually causes renal failure, manifested as decreased urine output (until oliguria or anuria occurs) and progressive uremia that can alter the level of consciousness. The administration of parenteral fluids usually will not reverse this circulatory shutdown at this stage of illness and can potentially worsen cases of fluid overload as renal function decreases.[6]

Decreased Levels of Consciousness

As patients approach death, most will have increased periods of drowsiness or lethargy, sometimes leading to coma. They may spend a large portion of the day asleep and will only interact with family and friends briefly before drifting back to sleep. When awake, the patient may speak very little, appear confused, or stare blankly into space with very little recognition of familiar people. Generally it is advisable to suggest to family members that a patient can still hear and feel their presence even after he or she stops talking and encourage them to talk softly to the patient, telling him or her any important things they would regret not saying. Situations involving family discord, including discussions of sensitive topics or arguing among family members, should be explicitly avoided in the presence of the patient. Families should be told that a patient might be awake or speak for brief periods of time and then go back to sleep. Progressively deeper and fluctuating levels of consciousness may be the final phases of a terminal delirium.

Agitation

Mild restlessness in dying patients may respond to turning, soft music, or gentle reassurance. On rare occasions, patients can become severely agitated immediately before death and require urgent treatment. (See section 5A (p. 91) for guidance about treating agitated delirium.) This distress could be due to potentially correctable problems such as stool impaction, a full bladder, or the inability to swallow analgesics. Distress also could be caused by an agitated terminal delirium that is not reversible and will require sedating medications. The development of an agitated terminal delirium can be a true crisis for families and should be treated as a palliative care emergency to be addressed quickly by the care team (see section 5A).

Incontinence

Nearly all patients will experience periods of incontinence of both urine and stool, particularly as a patient becomes bedbound and sphincter control gradually is lost. Incontinence can be distressing to family caregivers. They should be adequately prepared with absorbent pads, cleaning products, and creams to soothe irritated skin. Demonstrating how to clean and change a bedbound patient can be helpful. When urinary retention causes discomfort or incontinence creates severe skin breakdown or necessitates frequently changing or moving the patient, urinary catheters sometimes help. For patients with delirium, however, use of a catheter can worsen agitation. A bedpan or bedside commode initially is useful for patients with impaired mobility but is only effective when a patient has sphincter control and an awareness of the need to use the toilet.

Patients with diarrhea can be a particular challenge, and careful attention initially should focus on a review of medications. Simple adjustments in drugs previously needed to counteract opioid-induced constipation are effective in relieving symptoms of diarrhea. Patients actually may have worsening constipation or urinary retention that can cause "overflow" urinary incontinence or diarrhea. Abdominal and rectal examinations may be indicated to properly assess the etiology. Infrequently, patients may benefit from the use of a rectal drainage tube when there is a profuse amount of diarrhea. For many patients, decreased food and fluid intake combined with progressive loss of renal function and bowel motility reduce or eliminate incontinent episodes in the last days and hours prior to death. Family caregivers often are the first to notice these changes, so they should be educated about them and instructed to alert other members of the care team when they occur.

Changes in Breathing

For all patients, the dying process eventually involves noticeable changes in respiratory patterns. Breathing often becomes shallow and mixed with increasing periods of apnea, which can sometimes appear as "breath holds" or extend over several minutes, making it look like the patient has already died. The Cheyne-Stokes pattern of irregular respirations (ie, alternating periods of hypopnea, apnea, and tachypnea) can be distressing to the observer but also represents significant neurological changes and the progression of the disease into the terminal stage. Often families worry that a patient may be uncomfortable or suffocating and need early education regarding these expected changes in breathing patterns. Tachypnea does not necessarily indicate that a patient is uncomfortable. Oxygen usually is not beneficial, although some patients and families may find it psychologically comforting. Opioids or benzodiazepines are appropriate to manage any perception of breathlessness (see section 3B [p. 47]). A few last reflexive breaths may indicate the impending moment of death or follow the cessation of cardiac function.

Loss of Ability to Close Eyes

Changes in the orbit surrounding the eye, including the loss of fat and fluid, cause the eyes to fall posteriorly into the orbital sockets and leave the eyelids partially open. Patients blink less, and caregivers can become distressed by their loved ones seemingly staring blankly into space, even during periods of sleep. It is important to explain to the family that these changes are common and to attempt to maintain moisture on the conjunctiva by applying ophthalmologic lubricants or artificial tears several times a day.

Near-Death Awareness

Sometimes a dying person appears to be able to describe what the experience of dying is like; seemingly he or she may know when death is approaching or express what they need for a peaceful death.[9] Information about these experiences largely comes from anecdotes reported by families and healthcare professionals. The language patients use to communicate this death awareness may be symbolic, and the family members or caregivers may become frustrated or fearful with this type of discussion. Distinguishing between near-death awareness and delirium can be difficult (patients may indicate seeing and speaking to dead relatives), and palliative care professionals should listen attentively and allow families to derive their own interpretation or meaning from the experience.[9] Support from the interdisciplinary care team is crucial at these times. These experiences may be an important part of attaining meaningful spiritual and life closure for the patient and family and also can have strong influences (positive or negative) on the subsequent grief and bereavement experienced by caregivers following the patient's death.

Sites of Care

At times, the last hours or days of care may become overwhelming for family caregivers, especially if there are rapidly evolving symptom management needs such as worsening pain, dyspnea, vomiting, or agitation.

For patients cared for at home, a back-up plan always should be considered in advance of any unforeseen crisis. Home hospice services offer significant support and 24-hour access to hospice nurses by phone for advice. Some home hospice programs can augment traditional home health aide assistance with up to 24 hours of continuous skilled nursing care or inpatient level care per day for actively dying patients with persistent acute symptom management needs. Many hospice agencies also provide families with an emergency "comfort kit" containing many of the medications routinely needed for the last hours of care (eg, opioids, benzodiazepines, antiemetics, and an anticholinergic).

Despite the comprehensiveness of these services, they may not be adequate for all patients being cared for at home if a care crisis emerges. In such circumstances, some patients may need to be transferred to a hospital, an inpatient palliative care unit, or a hospice facility for the most effective acute symptom management and family support. Care coordination and communication during these transfers between sites of care is critical to ensure the least disruption possible to the patient and family. This communication involves emergency medical services (transfer of advance directives and DNR orders), nursing staff (both during the transfer and at the receiving sites of care), hospice providers, and the family. Some caregivers may feel defeated if they are unable to honor loved ones' requests to die at home, therefore it is important to provide as much reassurance and support as possible during these transitions.[10,11]

When Death Occurs

Preparation of family caregivers also should include a discussion about the steps to take after death occurs. For hospice patients who remain at home, families should be instructed to not call 911 when death occurs; instead, the hospice care team should be contacted directly. Ideally families already will have been planning arrangements with a funeral home. After the patient's death, the clinician pronouncing the patient should confirm that death has occurred, express condolences to the family for their loss, and ask the family if they have any additional questions. Family members should be allowed to spend as much time as desired with the patient; this is particularly important in hospitals and nursing homes, where often there is a sense of urgency to have the body removed and the room cleaned after a patient has died. Allow time and space for immediate grief reactions. Even when expected, initial emotional reactions can be intense. Each moment immediately after a patient's death is important in the bereavement process.

9B | Grief and Bereavement

Grief is a process that occurs in response to a loss. In palliative care, the losses tend to occur in association with a debilitating illness and include the loss of life, function, purpose, independence, home, dignity, and loved ones. This section will focus on the grief surrounding the dying process.

Anticipatory grief is experienced both by patients and loved ones before death occurs. While looking over the course of their life, patients may regret what they consider bad choices or strained relationships. They also may try to come to terms with leaving loved ones and the loss of a future they had envisioned for themselves. For family and friends, anticipatory grief involves preparing for a future without the patient. They may feel guilt over past conflicts. Expressing forgiveness, thanks, love, and farewell often are the themes predominating this phase of grief.[12]

Normal grief encompasses a wide range of experiences.[13] Although there can be common elements to the grieving process (eg, disbelief, yearning, anger, acceptance), these do not occur in any specific order and some may not occur at all. Grief may have certain triggers, such as the anniversary of the death, holidays, or reminders of the deceased. Common grief reactions include

- somatic symptoms
- sleep and appetite disturbances
- memory loss and impaired concentration
- social withdrawal and disinterest in prior activities
- a sense of the presence of the deceased person
- auditory or visual hallucinations

- questioning of spiritual/religious beliefs
- emotional reactions such as relief, numbness, helplessness, self-reproach, sadness, guilt, or despair.

Distinguishing a normal grief reaction from depression can be complicated because sadness, guilt, thoughts of death, and psychomotor retardation can be a normal part of grief.[13] Asking the survivor, "Do you feel depressed?" or "Are you able to experience any kind of enjoyment?" can be the initial step in screening for clinical depression.[14] This dialogue should take place before initiating referrals to mental health professionals or antidepressant therapies.

Complicated grief, which occurs in 10% to 20% of survivors, is a prolonged and pathological grieving process that includes the experiences listed above. However, although the sense of loss will never be completely gone, the intensity of uncomplicated grief usually abates over time. Intense grieving that persists for longer than 6 months may be a sign of complicated grief, especially if these symptoms cause marked disruption in social or work life. Often, the bereaved person may seem to be stuck in one of the stages of grieving mentioned above. Specific markers for complicated grief include

- yearning for the deceased to a distressing or disruptive degree
- trouble accepting death
- inability to trust others
- a high degree of bitterness or anger
- difficulty forming new relationships
- feeling detached or emotionally numb
- feeling that life is empty or meaningless.

Bereavement refers to the period after a loss during which grief is experienced and mourning occurs. The amount of time spent in bereavement will depend on a wide range of factors, including how attached the individual was to the person who died, the circumstances of the death, and the individual's other coping mechanisms and supports.

Mourning is the process by which people adapt to a loss. In addition to individual factors, mourning also is influenced by cultural customs, rituals, and social rules about coping with a loss. If a patient comes from a culture with which the treating team is unfamiliar, it is useful to have the family teach the team about their mourning practices so they can be honored and supported.

Traumatic death, death of a child, death with symptoms that may have been difficult to control, and unexpected or sudden death of a loved one can put survivors at increased risk for complicated grief, as can a history of mental health disorders or substance abuse. Recent losses of other loved ones put the bereaved at increased risk, as well. Differences in cultural traditions surrounding the grieving process must be taken into account before a determination regarding complicated grief is made.

Although there is no simple formula for responding to grief and bereavement, the EASE tool provides some guidance for an initial approach.[15]

- **Educate** survivors about the wide variety of experiences in normal grief; validate their emotions and reactions while reminding them that everyone may have different reactions.
- **Assess** for common grief reactions, mental and physical health, and history of other losses.
- **Support** by listening actively, sending a condolence card, providing written materials about grief, encouraging discussion with friends and family, and identifying local support groups, if needed. Psychotherapy or other specialized interventions may be needed in cases of complicated grief.
- **Explore** which support methods work best for the bereaved individual. Do they prefer verbal or written communication about their experience? Which interventions seem to help, and which don't?

All hospice programs and many palliative care programs have formal support programs for bereaved family members. These programs are sufficient for most family members, who often work through their grieving through a mix of informal channels. It is important for clinicians to reevaluate survivors' grieving processes at follow-up visits and to systematically reach out to those at risk for complicated grief. If signs of complicated grief arise, or if there is any indication of the risk of suicide, referral to a specialist in grief counseling is indicated. Because the range of normal grieving is wide, it is important to not overnormalize or over-pathologize.[15,16] If in doubt about whether to refer a given family member to a specialist, discuss the potential of consultation or counseling with the at-risk family member and other family members, if appropriate, and further discuss the case with other palliative care team members and colleagues with expertise in grief and bereavement.

Further Discussion

1. Name three medications can be used to manage copious oral or respiratory secretions during the terminal period for patients.

2. How would you describe to caregivers the expected changes they will observe during the dying process?

3. How are urinary and fecal incontinence best managed at the end of life?

4. What are the common changes observed in respiratory patterns at the end of life?

5. What would you instruct family caregivers in the home to do at the time they suspect death has occurred?

6. What is expected with normal grief and bereavement? When does it become complicated grief?

7. What are the components of the EASE tool?

References

1. Christakis NA, Lamont EB. Extent and determinants of error in physicians' prognoses in terminally ill patients: prospective cohort study. *West J Med.* 2000;172(5):310-313.

2. Ellershaw J, Ward C. Care of the dying patient: the last hours or days of life. *BMJ.* 2003;326(7379):30-34.

3. Ferris FD, von Gunten CF, Emanuel LL. Competency in end-of-life care: last hours of life. *J Palliat Med.* 2003;6(4):605-613.

4. LeGrand SB, Tropiano P, Marx JD, Davis MP, Walsh D. Dying at home: emergency medications for terminal symptoms. *Am J Hosp Palliat Care.* 2001;18(6):421-423.

5. Bailey FA. Comfort care order set: last hours of life. In: FA Bailey. *The Palliative Response.* 2nd ed. Birmingham, AL: Menasha Ridge Press; 2005.

6. Bruera E, Hui D, Dalal S, et al. Parenteral hydration in patients with advanced cancer: a multicenter, double-blind, placebo-controlled randomized trial. *J Clin Oncol.* 2013;31(1):111-118.

7. Prommer E. Anticholinergics in palliative medicine: an update. *Am J Hosp Palliat Care.* 2013;30(5):490-498.

8. Wildiers H, Dhaenekint C, Demeulenaere P, et al; Flemish Federation of Palliative Care. Atropine, hyoscine butylbromide, or scopolamine are equally effective for the treatment of death rattle in terminal care. *J Pain Symptom Manage.* 2009;38(1):124-133.

9. Marchand L. Near death awareness. *Fast Facts and Concepts #118.* Milwaukee, WI: End of Life/Palliative Education Resource Center; 2009. www.eperc.mcw.edu/EPERC/FastFactsIndex/ff_118.htm. Accessed October 24, 2013.

10. Stajduhar KI, Davies B. Variations in and factors influencing family members' decisions for palliative home care. *Palliat Med.* 2005;19(1):21-32.

11. Topf L, Robinson CA, Bottorff JL. When a desired home death does not occur: the consequences of broken promises. *J Palliat Med.* 2013;16(8):875-880.

12. Byock I. *The Four Things That Matter Most: A Book About Living.* New York, NY: Free Press; 2004.

13. Casarett D, Kutner JS, Abrahm J. Life after death: a practical approach to grief and bereavement. *Ann Intern Med.* 2001;134(3):208-215.

14. Chochinov HM, Wilson KG, Enns M, Lander S. "Are you depressed?" Screening for depression in the terminally ill. *Am J Psychiatry.* 1997;154(5):674-676.

15. Carrington NA, Bogetz JF. Normal grief and bereavement: letters from home. *J Palliat Med.* 2004;7(2):309-323.

16. Zhang B, El-Jawahri A, Prigerson HG. Update on bereavement research: evidence-based guidelines for the diagnosis and treatment of complicated bereavement. *J Palliat Med.* 2006;9(5):1188-1203.

TEN

Special Considerations for Infants and Children

Pediatric palliative care has many similarities to adult palliative care, but there are some important differences to be aware of when treating children. This chapter provides pediatric-specific information to supplement each of the nine preceding chapters. It is intended not to stand alone but instead to be read in conjunction with the corresponding section of the adult text.

10A | Talking with Parents and Children About Palliative Care and Hospice

Introducing Palliative Care to Parents of Sick Children

All of the challenges associated with talking to adults about palliative care are magnified when talking to parents of sick children. As with adults, palliative care should be a part of the treatment plan for seriously ill children from the time of diagnosis throughout the course of the disease.[1] The approach to introducing palliative care to patients described in section 1C generally can be applied when speaking with parents of a sick child, but extra sensitivity may be needed, and an emphasis should be placed on providing palliative care along with life-prolonging and curative therapies.

The natural instinct of parents is to protect their children. This instinct can be heightened when a child is sick and vulnerable, sometimes causing parents to be defensive when palliative care is initially introduced. Parents are often fearful that accepting palliative care services means their child will lose access to curative and life-prolonging therapies, or that their child's care team will stop offering more aggressive therapeutic options. It is very important to ask open-ended questions that give parents an opportunity to express their concerns about palliative care so their misconceptions can be corrected.

Palliative care often is introduced as an added layer of support that supplements, rather than detracts from, the care the child is already receiving. Parents can be told that the goal is to manage their child's symptoms just as aggressively as his or her underlying disease. Practitioners also can explain that parents of sick children often are asked to make complex, difficult decisions about the medical care their child receives; in turn, the palliative care team is there to ensure that the family is provided all of the information they need, that they understand the information, that they have time to ask questions, and that they are supported in whatever choices they make. Because sick children often have medically complex circumstances, there may be multiple subspecialists involved in their care. The palliative care team also can help ensure that all of the child's providers are aware of the family's preferences and of the goals of care for the child.

Introducing Hospice to Parents of Sick Children

Introducing hospice can be difficult for providers because it forces everyone to address the very uncomfortable fact that the child might die. In modern society, the death of a child seems unnatural and can be more difficult to understand than the death of an elderly person. Frequently, children with palliative care needs and their families experience significant uncertainty concerning the trajectory of the child's disease and prognosis. They may have been through prior episodes in which the child seemed close to death but recovered. This disease trajectory, marked by multiple life-threatening exacerbations, can make determining when to refer a child to hospice more challenging than for an adult. It also can make it more difficult for families to make the decision to stop pursuing curative and life-prolonging therapies. In recognition of this, the Patient Protection and Affordable Care Act passed in 2010 includes a provision, section 2303, termed the "Concurrent Care for Children Requirement." The new provision requires state Medicaid programs to pay for concurrent curative/life-prolonging treatment and hospice services for children younger than 21 years who have a prognosis of 6 months or less if the disease runs its normal course.[2] Some private insurance companies may provide coverage for concurrent hospice and curative/life-prolonging therapies, but they are not required to do so. This change in the Medicaid hospice eligibility requirements has made it easier for many parents to accept hospice services without feeling that they are giving up on their child.

Introducing Hospice and Palliative Care to Children

Sick children often want to know what is happening with their disease and have ideas about what should be done. Some parents are supportive of including their child in honest communication about the disease progression, but others are concerned that this type of communication will cause their child unnecessary worry or take away their child's hope. In fact, not including children in the discussion and pretending that everything is fine often causes children to lose trust in their caregivers and feel more frightened and isolated.[3] In the majority of these situations, when parents' concerns about sharing information with their child are addressed and the parents feel supported and respected by the care team, a plan for communicating with the child about his or her disease can be established. Section 10G suggests approaches to situations in which parents are resistant to sharing medical information with their sick child.

When speaking with a child about his or her medical condition, begin by finding out what the child is experiencing. What does the child know about the disease? What does the child think is happening? Why does the child think this is happening? Find out what the child wants to know by allowing the child to set the pace of the conversation and to ask questions. Before answering, ask clarifying questions to ensure you understand what the child wants to know and why. When delivering information, use simple, developmentally appropriate language. In children younger than 8 years, avoid euphemisms because they can be confusing to these concrete thinkers. Be sure to stop and acknowledge emotional reactions with empathetic statements that validate the child's experience and help him or her feel supported. Some children may have difficulty communicating their thoughts and feelings verbally. In these situations, expressive therapies such as art, music, and play therapy can be extremely helpful in allowing a child to express emotions and giving therapists insight into how the child is experiencing his or her disease.[4-7]

10B | Pain Management

The assessment of a child's pain must be appropriate to his or her developmental age. When a child has reached a developmental level at which he or she is able to provide a self-report, this is the best method of pain assessment. When asking a child about his or her pain, it is important to use the child's word for pain. Children may use terms such as "owie" or "boo-boo" and may be confused by the word "pain." At the age of 3 years, children begin to develop the skills necessary for using a tool to rate the severity of their pain. By the age of 4 years, the majority of children are able to use a pain self-report tool. For children between the ages of 3 and 7 years, pain scales should consist of a limited number of choices (generally fewer than six) and concrete descriptors such as faces. There are several different faces scales that can be used with this age group, such as the Faces Pain Scale-Revised (**Figure 10.1**). Visual analog scales or the standard 0-to-10 verbal numeric scales (Figure 2.1 [p. 14]) can be introduced around the developmental age of 8 years.[8,9]

When a child is unable to report his or her pain, an observational tool should be used. Most tools have been validated in a specific patient population or under a specific circumstance. For example, many tools have been validated only in the postoperative period. There is no one tool that has been validated across the full range of children receiving palliative care. The Face, Legs, Activity, Cry, and Consolability (FLACC) Pain Assessment Tool is commonly used in pediatric palliative care. It was validated in children younger than 3 years who were hospitalized with a variety of disease processes (**Table 10.1**).[10] In the neonatal period, it is common to use pain scales specifically designed for neonates. The CRIES scale was validated as a postoperative pain assessment tool, but frequently is used in the neonatal intensive care unit setting to assess pain from a wide range of sources (**Table 10.2**).[11] When using observational pain assessment tools, keep in mind that physiological indicators of pain, such as changes in pulse, blood pressure, and oxygen saturation, may not be reliable indicators in critically ill children or children with chronic pain. Facial grimacing and crying also may be less reliable indicators of pain in chronically ill children. Because pain assessment can be challenging in children, the presence of pain should always be considered in children who are withdrawn, irritable, or not engaging in developmentally appropriate activities. Clinicians should partner with parents in performing pain assessments because parents are often able to detect subtle changes in their child's behavior that may indicate an increase in pain.

Figure 10.1 Faces Pain Scale-Revised (FPS-R)

In the following instructions, say "hurt" or "pain," whichever seems right for a particular child.

"These faces show how much something can hurt. This face [point to left-most face] shows no pain. The faces show more and more pain [point to each from left to right] up to this one [point to right-most face]—it shows very much pain. Point to the face that shows how much you hurt [right now]."

Score the chosen face 0, 2, 4, 6, 8, or 10, counting left to right, so '0' = 'no pain' and '10' = 'very much pain.' Do not use words like 'happy' and 'sad'. This scale is intended to measure how children feel inside, not how their face looks.

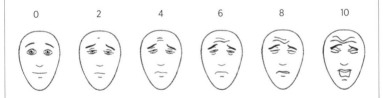

From Hicks CL, von Baeyer CL, Spafford P, van Korlaar I, Goodenough B. The Faces Pain Scale – Revised: toward a common metric in pediatric pain measurement. Pain. 2001;93:173-183. With the instructions and translations as found on the website: www.usask.ca/childpain/fpsr. This Faces Pain Scale-Revised has been reproduced with permission of the International Association for the Study of Pain® (IASP). The figure may NOT be reproduced for any other purpose without permission.

Table 10.1 FLACC Pain Assessment Tool[12]

SCORING CATEGORIES	0	1	2
Face	No particular expression or smile	Occasional grimace or frown, withdrawn, disinterested	Frequent-to-constant frown, quivering chin, clenched jaw
Legs	Normal position or relaxed	Uneasy, restless, tense	Kicking or legs drawn up
Activity	Lying quietly, normal position, moves easily	Squirming, shifting back and forth, tense	Arched, rigid, or jerking
Cry	No cry (awake or asleep)	Moans or whimpers; occasional complaint	Crying steadily, screams or sobs, frequent complaints
Consolability	Content, relaxed	Reassured by occasional touching, hugging, or being talked to; distractible	Difficult to console or comfort

From Merkel SI, Voepel-Lewis T, Shavevitz JR, Malviva S. The FLACC: a behavioral scale for scoring postoperative pain in young children. Pediatr Nurs. 1997;23(3):293-297. ©1997 Jannetti Publications, Inc. Reprinted with permission.

Table 10.2 CRIES Neonatal Postoperative Pain Measurement Tool

SCORING CATEGORIES	0	1	2
Crying	No	High-pitched	Inconsolable
Requires O_2 for oxygen saturation >95%	No	<30%	>30%
Increased vital signs	HR and BP ≤ or <preoperative value	HR or BP ↑ <20% of preoperative value	HR or BP ↑ >20% of preoperative value
Expression	None	Grimace	Grimace/grunt
Sleeplessness	No	The baby wakes at frequent intervals	The baby is awake continuously

Coding Tips for CRIES

Crying	The characteristic cry of pain is high-pitched.
	If there is no crying or it is not high-pitched . . . . score **0**
	If crying is high-pitched but the baby is easily consoled . . . . .score **1**
	If crying is high-pitched and the baby is inconsolable . . . . score **2**
Requires O_2 for oxygen saturation >95% *(Consider other causes of changes in oxygenation: atelectasis, pneumothorax, overse-dation, etc.)*	Look for changes in oxygenation. Babies experiencing pain manifest decreases in oxygenation as measured by TCO_2 or oxygen saturation.
	If no oxygen is required. . . . . score **0**
	If <30% O_2 is required . . . . .score **1**
	If >30% O_2 is required . . . . score **2**
Increased vital signs	Take blood pressure last, because this may wake the baby, making other assessments difficult.
	Use baseline preoperative parameters from a period free of stress. Multiply baseline HR by 0.2, then add this total to the baseline value to determine whether the HR is 20% faster.
	Do likewise for BP, using the mean value.
	If HR and BP are both either unchanged or less than at baseline . . . . score **0**
	If either HR or BP is <20% of baseline . . . . score **1**
	If either one is >20% from baseline. . . . . score **2**

continued

Table 10.2 CRIES Neonatal Postoperative Pain Measurement Tool continued

SCORING CATEGORIES	0	1	2
Expression	The facial expression most often associated with pain is a grimace characterized by a lowered brow, the eyes squeezed shut, a deepening of the nasolabial furrow, and open lips and mouth.		
	If no grimace is present. . . . . score **0**		
	If grimace alone is present . . . . score **1**		
	If grimace and a vocalization without crying (grunt) are present. . . . . score **2**		
Sleeplessness	This parameter is scored according to the infant's state during the preceding hour.		
	If the baby has been continuously asleep . . . . score **0**		
	If the baby has awoken at frequent intervals . . . . score **1**		
	If the baby has been awake continuously . . . . score **2**		

HR, heart rate; BP, blood pressure; $\uparrow$, increase; TCO_2, transcutaneous CO_2.

From Krechel SW, Bildner J. *CRIES: a new neonatal postoperative pain measurement score. Initial testing of validity and reliability.* Pediatric Anesthesia, 1995;5*(1):53–61. This neonatal pain assessment tool was developed at the University of Missouri–Columbia. ©1995 Krechel SW and Jo Bildner J. Reprinted with permission.*

Opioids

Opioids can be used safely and effectively to relieve many types of pain in children. It is important that chronic pain is treated with regularly scheduled doses of medication administered around the clock and that the child does not have to experience pain before receiving a dose of medication. Any child on scheduled doses of opioids should also have an as-needed (prn) dose available to treat breakthrough pain. Initial opioid dosages are always calculated based on a child's weight (see dosing guidelines in Table 2.1 [p.15]). Once an appropriate weight-based dosage is determined, the guidelines described in section 2A (p. 17) for opioid administration, titration, and conversion can be followed. Practitioners who do not prescribe opioids frequently should reference section 2D (p. 30) for dosing information pertinent to children and adults.

In addition to the guidelines in section 2A, it should be noted that codeine should not be used in children.[13] Codeine is metabolized to morphine by the cytochrome P450 enzyme, CYP2D6. Prior to being metabolized, codeine does not have an analgesic effect; rather, it is the morphine that provides the analgesia. There is wide genetic variability in the activity of CYP2D6, and deaths have been reported in children who are ultra-fast metabolizers of codeine.[14] Conversely, some children lack the enzyme to metabolize codeine to morphine and will not experience any pain relief from the medication. In one study, 35% of pediatric patients showed inadequate metabolism of codeine to morphine.[15]

Fentanyl and Methadone

Both methadone and transdermal fentanyl can be used in children, but they should be used with care as described in section 2B (p. 23). Methadone can be useful for treating pain in children because it is the only long-acting opioid available in liquid form. In the treatment of neuropathic pain, it has the additional benefit of acting not only as an agonist at the opioid receptors but also as an antagonist at the N-methyl D-aspartate receptors. Transdermal fentanyl can be appealing for use in children because it provides long-acting pain relief without the child having to swallow an oral medication. It is important to note that transdermal fentanyl should never be started without first titrating and achieving good pain control with a short-acting opioid. Children should be on at least an equivalent of 30 mg of oral morphine before starting a 12.5-mcg fentanyl patch.

Treatment of Acute Pain Crisis

Young children lack the cognitive maturity to understand why they are having pain and that the medications used to treat their pain take time to work. If pain medications are not titrated quickly, children may lose confidence in the medications and be resistant to taking them in the future. When a child is having an acute pain crisis it should be viewed as an emergency, and a provider should stay at the child's bedside managing the situation until the pain is under control (see section 2C [p. 29] for recommendations on managing an acute pain crisis).

General Opioid Caveats

In infants aged 6 months and younger, the starting opioid dose must be decreased to 25% to 33% of the usual starting dose. This dose adjustment is needed because infants have immature liver function, decreased clearance by the kidneys, a high ratio of body water to fat, reduced levels of circulating albumin and glycoprotein, and a larger portion of their body mass is made up of highly perfused tissues, such as in the brain, heart, and viscera. Also, reduced ventilatory response to low O_2 and high CO_2 can predispose infants to inadequate gas exchange and respiratory depression.[16]

In children, it is particularly important to be thoughtful about the route and frequency of medication administration. Being familiar with all of the possible routes of administration for each medication and choosing the route that is most appropriate for the child and the situation can have significant positive effects on the child's quality of life by minimizing the frequency and burden of medication administration. Whenever possible, the oral route is preferable. It is cost effective, allows for easy titration, does not require advanced skills to administer, and generally is less frightening to children than routes that involve needle sticks or suppositories. Although the oral route is preferable, children may have difficulty swallowing pills and may dislike the taste of liquid medications. Therefore, liquid medications, especially opioids, which have a particularly bad taste in liquid form, should be flavored to make them as palatable as possible. For children who need sustained-release opioids but cannot swallow tablets, a sustained-release morphine capsule that can be opened is available. The pellets within the capsules cannot be crushed or chewed, but they will maintain their sustained release properties when mixed with applesauce and swallowed. The pellets from the Kadian capsule also can be administered through a 16-French gastric tube.

For a whole range of reasons, including a child's preference, aspiration risk, gastrointestinal tract dysfunction, and pain crisis necessitating fast-acting medications, an administration route other than oral may be needed. Other routes to consider include intravenous (IV), which may be preferred by children who have permanent or semiperminent venous access, subcutaneous (SC), rectal, transdermal, transmucosal, epidural, or intrathecal. In general, the intramuscular route should be avoided because it is painful and may cause children to refuse future dosages of pain medication.

Addiction and Dependence

One might not expect parents to be concerned about addiction when opioids are suggested to treat pain in a child with palliative care needs, but it is a common concern. Parents often do not report this concern unless they are directly asked about it, but fear of addiction can be a major barrier to parents' willingness to allow their child's pain to be treated with opioids. However, there is no evidence that the appropriate use of opioids in children receiving palliative care leads to addiction.

When prescribing opioids and other controlled substances to children, the provider should be aware of any members of the child's household who have current or past addiction issues. The presence of members of the household with addiction issues does not prohibit the use of opioids to treat a child's pain, but in these situations, a plan should be instituted to avoid diversion of the child's medications. Lock boxes may be used in the home to secure medications, and a written pain contract or partnership agreement may be needed. Section 2E (p. 32) contains additional information on addiction and dependence.

Adjuvant Analgesia, Procedural Methods for Pain Relief, and Nonpharmacologic Methods

Along with opioids, adjuvant analgesics and procedural methods of pain relief can be used in children (see sections 2F [p. 34] and 2G [p. 35] respectively). **Table 10.3** includes several adjuvant medications that can be used in children, including acetaminophen, nonsteroidal anti-inflammatories, tricyclic antidepressants, gabapentin, baclofen, and glucocorticoids. Other adjuvants such as ketamine and lidocaine have been used in children, but a palliative medicine physician should be consulted if these medications are needed. Nonpharmacologic pain management techniques also can be effective in children. These

Table 10.3 Select Medications Used in Pediatric Palliative Medicine

DRUG	ROUTE	PEDIATRIC DOSAGE (MG/KG/DOSE, UNLESS BOLDED)	INTERVAL FOR ROUTINE DOSING BASED ON HALF-LIFE (HOURS)	MAXIMUM DOSAGE	COMMENTS
Nonopioid Analgesics (fever, mild pain)					
Acetaminophen	PO, PR, IV	10–15	4–6	75 mg/kg/day or 3 g/day	Rectal absorption variable IV form approved for children 2 years and older
Ibuprofen	PO	5–10	6–8	40 mg/kg/day or 3.2 g/day	Anti-inflammatory
Naproxen	PO	5–10	8–12	1 g/day	Anti-inflammatory Age older than 2 years
Opioid Analgesics (moderate to severe pain, dyspnea; titrate dosage to effect; for infants younger than 6 months, start at one-quarter to one-third of the recommended dosage). See Table 2.1 for more information.					
Benzodiazepines (agitation, anxiety, insomnia)					
Clonazepam	PO	0.005–0.01	8–12	0.1–0.2 mg/kg/day >10 years: 20 mg/day	Long-acting Titrate by 10%–25% every 2 or 3 days
Diazepam	PO, IV	0.04–0.2	6–12	<5 years: 5 mg/dose >5 years: 10 mg/dose	Medium-acting
Lorazepam	PO, SL, PR, IV, SC	0.02–0.05	4–12	Anxiety/Agitation: 2 mg/dose Seizures: 4 mg/dose	Medium-acting Useful for anticipatory nausea

continued

Table 10.3 Select Medications Used in Pediatric Palliative Medicine *continued*

DRUG	ROUTE	PEDIATRIC DOSAGE (MG/KG/DOSE, UNLESS BOLDED)	INTERVAL FOR ROUTINE DOSING BASED ON HALF-LIFE (HOURS)	MAXIMUM DOSAGE	COMMENTS
Prokinetic Antiemetic					
Metoclopramide	PO, IV, SC	0.1–0.2	6	0.8 mg/kg/day or 15 mg/dose	For nausea from gastic stasis, drugs, or metabolic products May cause dystonia
Antihistamines (nausea, vomiting, pruritis)					
Diphenhydramine	PO, IV, SC	0.5–1	4–8	50 mg/dose	Can relieve dystonia from phenothiazines or haloperidol
Hydroxyzine	PO, IM	0.5–1	4–6	100 mg/dose	SC and IV are contraindicated and not recommend under any circumstance
Neuroleptics (nausea, vomiting, delirium)					
Haloperidol	PO, IV, SC, IM	0.01–0.025	8–12	0.15 mg/kg/day	Age older than 3 years For delirium or nausea May cause dystonia
Prochlorperazine	PO, PR	0.1–0.15 or **2.5 mg/dose**	6–8	20 mg/day	Age older than 2 years May cause dystonia
Serotonin (5-HT₃) Receptor Antagonists (nausea, vomiting)					
Ondansetron	PO	0.15	8–12	8 mg/dose	Alternative dose by age: 4–11 years, use 4 mg every 8 hours; 12 years and older, use 8 mg every 8 hours
	IV, SC	0.1–0.15	8–12		

continued

Table 10.3 Select Medications Used in Pediatric Palliative Medicine *continued*

DRUG	ROUTE	PEDIATRIC DOSAGE (MG/KG/DOSE, UNLESS BOLDED)	INTERVAL FOR ROUTINE DOSING BASED ON HALF-LIFE (HOURS)	MAXIMUM DOSAGE	COMMENTS
Corticosteroids (anti-inflammatory, nausea, vomiting, pain, anorexia)					
Dexamethasone	PO, IV, SC	Anti-inflammatory: 0.08-0.3 **mg/kg/day** Antiemetic: 0.1 mg/kg/dose Brain-tumor associated cerebral edema: initial loading dose: 1-2 **mg/kg** maintenance dose: 1-2 **mg/kg/day**	6-24 6-24	16 mg/day 50-100 mg 16 mg/day	May cause mood swings, psychosis, or long-term side effects Not typically used on prn basis Adjust downward as clinically indicated.
Anticholinergics (secretions)					
Scopolamine	Transder-mal	1 patch (1.5 mg)	Every 3 days		Age older than 12 years Place behind ear. Movement-related nausea or troublesome secretions
Glycopyrrolate	PO	0.04-0.1	4-8	Max 1-2 mg/dose PO, 8 mg/day	
	IV, SC	0.004-0.01	4-8		
Psychostimulants (opioid sedation, depression)					
Methylphenidate	PO	0.1 mg/kg/dose or 2.5-5 **mg/dose**	Morning and noon	0.5 mg/kg/day or 60 mg/day	Can exacerbate anxiety or agitation Avoid use in patients with pre-existing structural cardiac abnormalities or other serious heart problems

continued

Table 10.3 Select Medications Used in Pediatric Palliative Medicine *continued*

DRUG	ROUTE	PEDIATRIC DOSAGE (MG/KG/DOSE, UNLESS BOLDED)	INTERVAL FOR ROUTINE DOSING BASED ON HALF-LIFE (HOURS)	MAXIMUM DOSAGE	COMMENTS
Tricyclic Antidepressants (neuropathic pain)					
Amitriptyline	PO	0.1-2 Start at 0.1 mg/kg, give at bedtime and titrate slowly	Single or divided doses	5 mg/kg/day 200 mg/day (Maximum dosing for depression)	Age older than 6 years Antidepressant dose higher than analgesic dose Increase dose gradually every few days. Most anticholinergic Risk of QT prolongation with higher doses and/or drug interactions
Desipramine	PO	25-50 **mg/day** (initial dose) May gradually increase if needed	Single or divided doses	150 mg/day	Age older than 12 years Increase dose gradually every few days. Risk of QT prolongation with higher dose and/or drug interactions
Nortriptyline	PO	1-3 **mg/kg/day**	Divided doses	Child: 10-20 mg/day Adolescent: 30-50 mg/day Adult: 75-100 mg/day	Older than 6 years Increase dose gradually every few days by 0.2 mg/kg/day. Risk of QT prolongation with higher dose and/or drug interactions
ANTICONVULSANTS (NEUROPATHIC PAIN)					
Gabapentin	PO	3-5 **mg/kg** (initial dose)	3 times daily (see comment)	300-mg initial dose 3,600 mg/day	First 3 days: give 1 dose on first day, 2 doses on second day, 3 doses on third day Titrate slowly.

continued

Table 10.3 Select Medications Used in Pediatric Palliative Medicine *continued*

DRUG	ROUTE	PEDIATRIC DOSAGE (MG/KG/DOSE, UNLESS BOLDED)	INTERVAL FOR ROUTINE DOSING BASED ON HALF-LIFE (HOURS)	MAXIMUM DOSAGE	COMMENTS
Miscellaneous					
Octreotide	SC, IV	0.001–0.01 **mg/kg/dose** (1-10 **mcg/kg/day**) or 1-2 **mcg/kg/dose**	Continuous or 2-3 times daily	1,500 mcg/day	Antisecretory agent for bowel obstruction Titrate up by 0.3 mcg/kg/dose every 3 days. Limited data in children
Baclofen	PO	2.5-5 **mg/dose** (2-7 years) 5 **mg/dose** (Older than 7 years)	3 times daily	40 mg/day (2-7 years) 60 mg/day (8 years and older) 80 mg/day (adult)	Age older than 2 years Titrate dose up every 3 days For nerve pain or spasticity Watch for withdrawal symptoms—seizure, anxiety, hallucinations

IM, intramuscular; IV, intravenous; PO, by mouth; PR, per rectum; SC, subcutaneous; SL, sublingual.

From Micromedex® Healthcare Series [Internet database]. Greenwood Village, CO: Thomson Healthcare; Robertson J, Shilkofski N. (Eds.), Harriet Lane Handbook: A Manual for Pediatric House Officers, 19th ed., Philadelphia: Mosby; 2011; and Takemoto CK, Hodding JH, Kraus DM. Pediatric & Neonatal Dosage Handbook, 20th ed. Hudson, OH, Lexi-Comp, Inc; 2013.

techniques should not be substituted for pharmacologic management, but whenever possible they should be used in conjunction with pharmacologic management. Nonpharmacologic pain management techniques are listed in Table 2.4 (p. 40).

10C | Dyspnea

Dyspnea refers to the subjective phenomenon of feeling short of breath, and its severity can be evaluated only by a self-report. There are few dyspnea scales that have been validated in children. One scale was validated in hospitalized children as young as 6 years with asthma.[17] Another scale, the Dalhousie Dyspnea Scale, was found to be valid in children 8 to 18 years of age with cystic fibrosis and asthma (**Figure 10.2**).[18] When a child reaches the developmental age of 8 years (the age at which the Dalhousie Dyspnea Scale becomes appropriate), visual analog and 1-to-10 verbal numeric scales also can be used to assess the severity of dyspnea. The evaluation of dyspnea in young children can be challenging because there are no validated dyspnea scales for children younger than 6 years, but many practitioners use a verbal descriptor scale consisting of a series of words. The child is asked a question such as "Do you have trouble breathing not at all, a little bit, a lot, or the most?" Although there is minimal evidence of the reliability and validity of verbal descriptor scales and there are no standard descriptors, they often are used because a better alternative doesn't exist. Once a tool for assessing dyspnea has been chosen, it should be used consistently so the child becomes comfortable with the scale and the severity of dyspnea can be accurately compared over time. If a verbal descriptor scale is used, the same descriptors should be used by all involved practitioners each time the child's dyspnea is assessed.

Figure 10.2 Dalhousie Dyspnea Scale

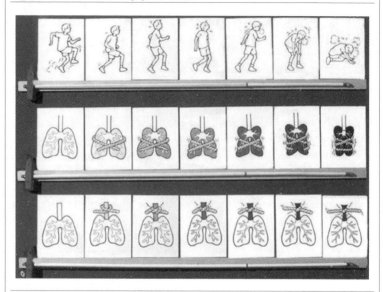

From McGrath PJ, Pianosi PT, Unruh AM, Buckley CP. Dalhousie dyspnea scales: construct and content validity of pictorial scales for measuring dyspnea. BMC Pediatr. 2005;5:33. ©2005 *BioMed Central Ltd. Reprinted with permission.*

Etiology

Common etiologies of dyspnea in children receiving palliative care include malignancies, cystic fibrosis, congenital or acquired cardiac disease, neuromuscular diseases such as spinal muscular atrophy, muscular dystrophies, pneumonia, and excessive secretions. In a study of 515 children who received palliative care consults at six different pediatric hospitals, more than 20% had dyspnea. The study also found that 10.1% of the children had respiratory disease that was significant enough to result in the placement of a tracheostomy.[19]

General Treatment Measures, Dyspnea in the Imminently Dying, and Continual Reassessment

The approach to the treatment of dyspnea in children is the same as that for adults, as described in sections 3B (p. 47), 3C (p. 54), and 3D (p. 55). The underlying etiology of the child's dyspnea always should be identified and disease-directed treatment consistent with the goals of care should be implemented. For symptomatic treatment of dyspnea, both pharmacologic and nonpharmacologic interventions should be implemented concurrently. As in adults, opioids can be used safely and effectively to suppress the awareness of the sensation of shortness of breath, and anxiolytics can be used to treat the anxiety that frequently accompanies dyspnea. In opioid-naïve children, a low dose of morphine (0.15 mg/kg/dose PO or 0.05 mg/kg/dose IV for children older than 6 months) often is effective, but it is important to titrate opioids appropriately until the dyspnea is controlled. If the dyspnea is severe, it should be viewed as a palliative care emergency and a provider may need to stay at the child's bedside to titrate medications. In these situations, the IV or SC routes of administration are preferred to achieve faster symptom relief. If the dyspnea is not expected to improve, scheduled opioid doses or a continuous opioid infusion should be started to prevent recurrent symptoms and suffering.

When a child is unable to report dyspnea but has labored breathing, it should be referred to as respiratory distress instead of dyspnea. Opioids remain the first-line therapy in these situations and should be appropriately titrated until nonverbal signs of distress, such as facial grimacing, resolve.

When opioids are being used to treat dyspnea at the end of life, family members and care providers may be concerned that the medication will hasten the patient's death, particularly if the patient previously has not been on opioids. The provider treating the dyspnea should address this potential concern by asking the family if they have any concerns about the medications being given. The provider also should speak with the care team to assess for any other concerns. It is not uncommon for the nurse who administers the final dose of an opioid prior to a child's death to feel that the medication killed the child. If the nurse's concern is not addressed, it can lead to undertreatment of other patients in the future. The prescribing provider should speak with the care team separately from the family to allow them to openly express their concerns. It should be explained gently to both the family and the care team that the child is dying because of his or her underlying disease, and that it is important to treat symptoms that are causing suffering during the dying process. It should also be explained that appropriately dosed and titrated opioids rarely hasten death in children.

Respiratory Secretions

As in adults, respiratory secretions at the end of life are common in children and can be very distressing to caregivers. Secretion management, as described in section 3E (p. 55), should be implemented. Repositioning and postural drainage can be effective, but in most cases, anticholinergic medications should be started as soon as the pooling of secretions in the tracheobronchial tree is noted on a physical exam. Anticholinergics typically are more effective when they are started early rather than after the sounds created by the pooled secretions are heard easily at the bedside without a stethoscope. Glycopyrrolate is a good option for children. It does not cross the blood-brain barrier as other anticholinergic medications do, so the child's risk of delirium is not increased. Also, it is easy to dose in children of any age. When glycopyrrolate is given intravenously or subcutaneously, a dose of 0.01 mg/kg/dose can be started every 4 hours scheduled or prn. However, it is important to note that glycopyrrolate is not absorbed well in the stomach. For this reason, when given through a gastric tube, the dose is 10 times the IV or SC dose (0.1 mg/kg/dose). Scopolamine patches can be used in children older than 12 years, and hyoscyamine can be used in children as young as 2 years.

10D | Gastrointestinal Symptoms

Common Oral Symptoms

In the midst of caring for complex palliative care patients, it is easy to overlook assessment of the oral cavity. Regular assessment for oral pain, dryness, and taste disorders can help identify issues early so that attempts can be made to minimize or prevent discomfort. Common oral symptoms and their treatments are reviewed in section 4A (p. 61). Twice daily cleaning of the teeth and gums with a fluoride toothpaste is basic prevention. If this is not possible, mouth-care sponges can be dipped in mouthwash and used to clean the teeth and gums.

Basic mouth care is something that patients and family members can be easily taught. Having something active to do for their child may give parents a sense of control, particularly as a child approaches death and there is little they are able to control. As the end of life approaches and the child stops eating and drinking, family members should be instructed to dip mouth-care sponges in water and use them to moisten their child's mouth on a regular basis. Caregivers also should ensure that the child's lips stay moist.

Dysphagia

Dysphagia is very common in children receiving palliative care, and its management varies depending on the goals of care. In situations when placing a feeding tube is inconsistent with the goals of care, consulting with a speech pathologist or specialized occupational therapist may be helpful. The therapist can evaluate the patient and teach the family ways to minimize aspiration, such as appropriately positioning the child during feeding and ensuring that the consistency of the food offered is suitable. Specialized equipment, such as a feeding chair, also may be recommended. In some cases, if the child's condition is not progressive, the therapists may provide exercises to improve coordination and muscle strength.

Artificial Nutrition and Hydration

Providing nutrition and hydration through nasogastric tubes (NG), nasojejunal tubes (NJ), and gastrostomy tubes (G) is very common in children receiving palliative care. In one study of 515 patients who received inpatient palliative care consults at six different pediatric hospitals, 68.2% of children were noted to have some type of feeding tube.[19] There are very little data in the pediatric population to help clinicians identify which children will have life prolongation or improved quality of life after placement of a G tube. However, adult data potentially may be generalized to children with advanced cancer, advanced organ failure, and persistent vegetative state (see table 4.1 [p. 68]). There are few studies that have analyzed the effects of NG, NJ, and G tube placement in neurologically impaired children, such as those with neurodegenerative conditions, neuromuscular conditions, and cerebral palsy. In some children, the placement of a feeding tube may enable weight gain and increase the ease of feeding and medication delivery.[20,21] Potential complications of G-tube placement include the risks associated with surgery and anesthesia; postsurgical complications, such as localized peritonitis and other infections; and long-term complications, such as local pain, skin breakdown, cellulitis, formation of granulation tissue, and leakage of gastric contents. If the benefits of G-tube placement are unclear in a particular patient, a time-limited trial of NG tube feeds can be performed to help determine whether G-tube placement will meet the patient's goals.

In general, a G tube is placed for long-term use, and NG or NJ tubes are used as short-term interventions. In neurologically impaired children with a poor prognosis, NG tubes can be used for many months if the child's parents understand the benefits and burdens and do not want their child to undergo surgery for G tube placement. The major complication associated with prolonged NG tube use is sinusitis. To minimize this risk, the NG tube should be replaced and the nostril in which the tube is placed rotated every month. There also is a risk of the tube being mistakenly placed in the lung. It can be fatal if feedings are administered through a misplaced tube, so NG tube placement should be checked carefully to minimize the risk of this complication.

Nausea and Vomiting

Before determining a course of treatment for nausea and vomiting, it is important to try to identify the underlying cause of the symptom. Gastrointestinal, central nervous system, metabolic, psychological, and pharmacologic factors can all contribute (see Figure 4.1 [p. 73], which shows the pathophysiology of vomiting). Even if the underlying cause of the nausea cannot be reversed, understanding the cause can be helpful in targeting therapy appropriately. See section 4D (p. 72) for a description of the causes of nausea and vomiting and etiology-specific management.

When nausea is identified in a child, a scheduled dose of a medication selected based on the etiology of the child's nausea should be started. If the child cannot tolerate an oral medication, then the IV, SC, or rectal routes should be considered. When nausea is temporally associated with meals or seems to be related to slow gastric emptying, a prokinetic agent such as metoclopramide, can be very effective. Metoclopramide is a convenient option because it can be administered via oral, SC, or IV routes and can be used in a child of any age.

An antidopaminergic medication is a good choice when the suspected cause of the child's nausea is stimulation of the chemoreceptor trigger zone by drugs or metabolic products. Haloperidol has strong antidopaminergic effects and can be used in children older than 3 years of age. In addition to its prokinetic effects, metoclopramide also can be used for its antidopaminergic activity. There is a risk of an acute dystonic reaction when using antidopaminergic medications, however, so the smallest effective dose should be used. Tardive dyskinesia related to metocloprimide is rare in children but has been reported in the literature. The risk of tardive dyskinesia increases with prolonged use of metocloprimide. The risk of a dystonic-dyskinetic reaction to metoclopramide is greatest in girls between 12 and 19 years and was estimated in one study to be 1:5,000 in this demographic.[22] If extrapyramidal side effects do occur, they can be treated with 1 mg/kg of diphenhydramine.

Ondansetron, which is a serotonin antagonist at the 5-HT$_3$ receptor, is helpful for postsurgical and chemotherapy-induced nausea and vomiting. However, this class of medication often causes constipation. Steroids can be used for nausea and vomiting caused by increased intracranial pressure or partial bowel obstruction. Antihistamines, such as meclizine, hydroxyzine, and diphenhydramine, can be used when there is an inner-ear pathology or motion sickness. It is common for children to have anticipatory nausea and vomiting, which can be treated with a benzodiazepine. As in adults, octreotide can be used for intractable nausea and vomiting, particularly in the setting of bowel obstruction or severely decreased gastrointestinal motility. When nausea is difficult to manage, several medications from different classes may need to be combined.

Nonpharmacologic methods for treating nausea and vomiting should be implemented in conjunction with pharmacological treatments whenever possible (see section 4D [p. 72]). When anxiety is contributing to nausea, the child should be taught relaxation techniques such as self-hypnosis. If certain odors trigger nausea, aromatherapy can be used to mask the unpleasant smell. Acupuncture and acupressure also can be considered.[23]

Constipation

Constipation commonly is seen in the palliative care setting secondary to the use of constipating medications, such as opioids and ondansetron. Chronic constipation also is common in neurologically impaired children secondary to poor tone and immobility.

The evaluation for constipation can be more difficult in pediatric patients than in adults. Infants and young children have decreased transit time through the intestine. Transit time increases throughout childhood, resulting in gradually fewer stools each day. The normal number of bowel movements each day varies widely, particularly in infants, who can have as many as 10 stools a day, or if breast fed, may go several days without a bowel movement. Most young children have one to three bowel movements each day. Taking a good history, including the child's previous and current bowel patterns and the consistency of his or her stools, will be helpful in the identification of changes. If constipation is suspected, a rectal examination to evaluate for impaction should be conducted, unless this type of exam is contraindicated due to another condition, such as neutropenia. The fifth finger should be used for examination of smaller children.

Stool impaction in a child is managed the same way as for an adult (see section 4E [p. 80]). Mineral oil rectal liquid can be used in children as young as 5 years. For children younger than 5 years, a glycerin rectal solution can be used in place of mineral oil. After any hard, impacted stool is removed, a combination of oral agents and suppositories can be used until the patient's bowel movements become regular. After constipation has been relieved, a maintenance dose of an oral medication should be started to prevent future constipation.

When constipation is chronic, a scheduled oral medication should always be started. Suppositories and enemas can be used as needed as rescue medications. Stool softeners (docusate), stimulant laxatives (senna, bisacodyl, prune juice), or osmotic agents (polyethylene glycol, lactulose, sorbitol) all can be used. Psyllium and other fiber-based compounds should be avoided in children with less than optimal fluid intake, which is typically the case in very ill and dying children. As with adults, children should be started on a bowel regimen when opioids are initiated. In these cases, a stool softener typically is not effective on its own and if used should be combined with a stimulant.

Senna is a good stimulant laxative for children and is available in both tablet and liquid forms. Alternatively, it can be brewed as a tea. Senna can be used in children as young as 1 month. For children younger than 1 month, prune juice (1 mL/kg to 2 mL/kg) can be given once a day. Polyethylene glycol is commonly prescribed by pediatricians despite limited data on its use in children; doses of 0.25 g/kg/24 hours to 1.42 g/kg/24 hours in children as young as 6 months of age have been reported.[24] When a child weighs more than 20 kg, an adult dose of 17 g per day can be used. The advantage of polyethylene glycol is that it is tasteless and may be easier to administer because it can be mixed with any liquid the child enjoys. However, it must be mixed with 4 oz to 8 oz of liquid, depending on the dose, which may be a large volume for very sick children to drink. Lactulose and sorbitol require the child to take a smaller volume of medication, but the child may not like the excessively sweet taste of these medications.

When oral medications alone are not effective, suppositories may be used. Glycerin suppositories frequently are the first choice, particularly for infants and young children. If the full suppository is too large, it may be cut horizontally into slivers. When glycerin suppositories are not effective, bisacodyl suppositories can be used. The 10-mg suppository can be cut in half horizontally to provide a 5-mg dose for children younger than 2 years. A 5-mg to 10-mg dose can be used in children between the ages of 2 and 11 years, and children older than 11 years can receive a 10-mg dose.

10E | Depression, Anxiety, Delirium, and Fatigue

Depression and Anxiety

Depression and anxiety are common in chronically ill children, and their presence may exacerbate other symptoms, interfere with the child's adherence to treatment, and negatively impact medical outcomes. The appropriate treatment of these conditions can enhance the child's quality of life and may even improve the physician's ability to manage the child's underlying disease and associated symptoms. Assessment for depression and anxiety is similar for both children and adults (see section 5B [p. 100), but because establishing a diagnosis and making a treatment plan for children can be challenging, it is often helpful to involve a child and adolescent psychiatrist.

Children who are depressed may present slightly differently than depressed adults. They tend to experience more irritability and guilt and have more somatic complaints. They may regress, exhibiting behavior typically associated with a younger developmental age; seem apathetic; and not adhere to prescribed medical treatments.

When anxiety or depression is diagnosed, nonpharmacologic interventions should be initiated. Therapeutic interventions may reduce distress and help children find ways to express their feelings about their lives and illness. For some children, talk therapy may be effective, but many have difficulty expressing their feelings with words. Studies have suggested that cognitive behavioral therapy alone or in combination with antidepressants can be effective for the treatment of depression.[25] Although commonly used, there is less evidence in the literature to support the use of other nonpharmacologic interventions in the treatment of children with anxiety and depression. Interventions that can be considered include guided imagery, hypnosis, [26] relaxation,[26] play therapy,[4] bibliotherapy,[15] art therapy,[7] pet therapy,[27] and writing.

When pharmacologic treatments are needed, consider consulting a child and adolescent psychiatrist. When treating anxiety, remember that although benzodiazepines may be effective for short-term treatment, they should be used with caution because they can cause sedation, confusion, paradoxical agitation, and behavioral inhibition. Trials analyzing the treatment of depression in children with cancer have shown both citalopram and fluvoxamine to be well tolerated.[28,29] The use of tricyclic antidepressants for depression also has been reported in children.[30,31] Citalopram, fluvoxamine, and tricyclic antidepressants all have a US Food and Drug Administration black box warning of increased suicide risk in children, adolescents, and young adults with major depression or other psychiatric disorders. The use of low-dose stimulants has been reported as an alternative to these medications, particularly in children who have a prognosis of weeks to months. These medications should be used with caution, however, because they can exacerbate anxiety.[32]

Delirium

Delirium has been reported in children as young as 6 months of age and likely is an underrecognized condition in critically ill and dying children.[33] The definition, differential diagnosis, history, examination, and diagnostic work-up of delirium in children are similar to those in adults (see section 5A [p. 91]). When evaluating for delirium in young children, it is important to know that the inability to maintain attention may manifest in infants and toddlers as difficulty engaging with others, whereas in children, adolescents, and adults, it manifests as distractibility and an inability to focus. When orientation is tested in young, verbal children, it is important to remember that the children only can be expected to be oriented to person and place because they have not developed enough understanding of the days of the week or dates to be able to answer questions about time.[33]

When treating delirium, reversible causes should be identified and addressed and nonpharmacologic interventions initiated (see section 5A). When needed, antipsychotic medications can be used safely and effectively in children. As in adults, the first-line pharmacologic treatment for delirium in children generally is haloperidol. In one study of

40 children in the intensive care unit diagnosed with delirium, haloperidol and risperidone were both found to be safe and effective treatment choices.[34] Risperidone is typically not used in children younger than 9 years. Chlorpromazine is a more sedating antipsychotic than haloperidol and can be used if agitation cannot be controlled with haloperidol. When an antipsychotic agent other than haloperidol is needed, often it is best to consult with a child and adolescent psychiatrist. When using haloperidol, be aware of the risk of extrapyramidal side effects. If they occur, they can be treated with 1 mg/kg of diphenhydramine.

Benzodiazepines generally should not be used for the treatment of delirium because they can cause paradoxical agitation and worsen symptoms of delirium. One exception is irreversible delirium, particularly at the end of life. Under this circumstance, benzodiazepines are a reasonable choice.

Fatigue

Fatigue is the most frequent symptom experienced by children with cancer[35] and is also common in other children receiving palliative care. The evaluation of fatigue, differences between primary and secondary fatigue, and common causes of fatigue in palliative care patients are discussed in section 5C (p. 111). The first step in the management of fatigue in children is implementing nonpharmacologic interventions, such as counseling children and their parents on using energy-conservation strategies. These strategies include maintaining a consistent daily routine, prioritizing activities, and scheduling high-priority activities during the time of day when the child has the most energy. Attention also should be paid to ensuring adequate sleep and optimizing nutritional status to the extent that it is comfortable for the child. As described in chapter 5, secondary causes of fatigue should be treated if consistent with the goals of care (Table 5.8 [p. 113]).

Psychostimulants, such as methylphenidate, can be added if pharmacologic treatment of fatigue is needed.[36,37] However, these medications generally should be avoided in patients with seizure disorders, anxiety, agitation, hypertension, structural cardiac abnormalities, cardiomyopathy, and serious heart rhythm abnormalities.

10F | Spiritual, Religious, and Existential Suffering

A child's parents and close relatives heavily influence his or her spiritual and religious experience. When addressing spiritual, religious, and existential issues in the pediatric setting, it is particularly important to view the whole family as the unit of care. When parents are well supported during experiences that cause spiritual and existential suffering, they are better able to provide care and support to their sick child. Care and reassurance from parents can be critical as children try to make sense of their illness and its meaning. Chapter 6 should be reviewed and its contents applied when treating spiritual, religious, and existential suffering in sick children and their families.

One of the unique factors in addressing spiritual and religious issues in children is that a child's conceptual understanding of spirituality and religion evolves as the child develops cognitively and emotionally. Although each child is unique, James Fowler's Stages of Faith can give care providers a framework to help them anticipate a child's level of understanding of spirituality and religion at different ages and developmental stages. Fowler's work builds on Erik Erikson's stages of psychosocial development and Piaget's stages of cognitive development. **Table 10.4** shows stages of cognitive development based on the work of Piaget, the concept of death that corresponds to each level of cognitive development, the characteristics of the child's spirituality based on Fowler's work, and supportive interventions that can be helpful at each stage of development.

Just as with adults, children want to know that their lives mattered and that they will be remembered. They often are interested in creating a legacy. This can be done in many ways, including making a video, writing letters, or drawing pictures to leave with loved ones. A child also may want to designate certain people to receive their prized possessions.

Table 10.4 Stages of Development and Supportive Interventions

AGE	STAGE OF COGNITIVE DEVELOPMENT	CONCEPT OF DEATH	SPIRITUALITY	SUPPORTIVE INTERVENTIONS
Infancy: 0-2 years	• Sensorimotor • Experience of the world through sensory information • Limited conscious thinking • Limited language • Reality that is based on physical needs being met	• Death is perceived as separation or abandonment	• Undifferentiated • Faith reflects trust and hope in others • Need for sense of self-worth and love	• Provide maximum physical relief and comfort • Provide comfort through sensory input (eg, touching, rocking, sucking) • Provide comfort with familiar people and transitional objects (eg, toys)
Early Childhood: 2-6 years	• Stage of preoperational thought • Prelogical • Development of representational or symbolic language • Egocentric orientation • Magical thinking	• Death is reversible or temporary • May equate death with sleep • May believe they can cause death by their thoughts (eg, wishing someone would go away caused the death) • May not express personal emotion, but may associate death with the sorrow of others • May see death as a punishment	• Intuitive • Faith is fantasy-filled, imitative, and imaginative • Emphasis on participation in ritual	• Minimize the child's separation from usual caregivers (eg, parents) or provide reliable and consistent substitutes • Dispel misconceptions about death as punishment for bad thoughts or actions • Provide concrete information about the state of death (eg, a "dead person no longer breathes or eats")

continued

Table 10.4 Stages of Development and Supportive Interventions *continued*

AGE	STAGE OF COGNITIVE DEVELOPMENT	CONCEPT OF DEATH	SPIRITUALITY	SUPPORTIVE INTERVENTIONS
Middle Childhood: 7-12 years	• Stage of concrete operations • Logical • No abstract reasoning • Orientation is egocentric	• Death is irreversible but is unpredictable • Aware that death is personal and can happen to them • May have great interest in details • May be interested in what happens after death • Can understand the biologic essentials of death	• Mythic: takes on stories and beliefs of community • Faith is literal and concerns right and wrong • Connects ritual with personal identity	• Evaluate for fears of abandonment, destruction, or body mutilation • May benefit from specifics about the illness and treatments and reassurance that treatments are not punishments • Maintain the child's access to peers • Foster the child's sense of mastery and control
Adolescence and Adulthood: Older than 12 years	• Stage of formal operations • Development of abstract thought and advanced logical functions (eg, complex analogy, deduction)	• Death is irreversible, universal, and personal, but distant • Has the ability to develop natural, physiological, and theological explanations of death	• Approaches synthesis: more conventional • Formation of a personal faith, incorporating environment and experience • Evolution of a relationship with God or a higher power • Searches for meaning, purpose, hope, and the value of life	• Reinforce comfortable body image, self-esteem • Allow expression of anger • Provide privacy for the child • Support reasonable measures for the child to achieve independence • Maintain the child's access to peers • Consider peer support groups

Adapted and modified from Stevens MM. Psychological adaptation of the dying child. In: Doyle E, Hanks GWC, Cherny N, Calman K, eds. Oxford Textbook of Palliative Medicine. 3rd ed. London, England: Oxford University Press; 2005:799; Rando TA. Grief, Dying and Death: Clinical Implications for Caregivers. Champaign, IL: Research Press; 1984:385-39l; Fowler JW. Stages of Faith: The Psychology of Human Development and the Quest for Meaning. New York, NY: Harper Collins; 1981; and Himelstein BP, Hilden JM, Boldt AM, Weissman D. Pediatric palliative care. N Engl J Med. 2004;350:1752-1762. ©2004 Massachusetts Medical Society. Adapted with permission.

Ensuring that their child is remembered and finding meaning in their child's life, illness, and death is often a part of parents' spiritual journeys. Palliative care teams can help parents create legacy items such as hand- and footprints, hand sculptures, photographs, and videos. Families also may create rituals to remember their child or charitable events or funds in memory of their child.

10G | Goal Setting, Prognosticating, and Self-Care

Setting Patient-Centered Goals

The approach to goal setting described in chapter 7 should be reviewed and applied when speaking with the parents of a sick child. The unique piece of goal setting for children is determining when and how to involve the child in discussions and decision making. Some parents are open to allowing developmentally appropriate disclosure of medical information to their sick child. Other parents are concerned that providing information will cause their child unnecessary emotional pain and suffering and are extremely resistant to involving their child in goal setting.

The ultimate goal is to promote a safe environment in which families are supported in discussing difficult topics with children. In some circumstances, a child psychologist or specially trained therapist may be able to teach parents how to talk to their children about difficult subjects at a developmentally appropriate level and facilitate these conversations. As with adult patients, the individual child's desire to receive medical information needs to be assessed and respected. Children typically have questions about their disease. They feel changes in their bodies as their disease progresses and don't always know how to interpret the changes. They see emotional responses in the adults around them and wonder if they have done something to cause the emotion. When children perceive that asking questions about their disease will make their parents sad or in any way alienate them, they typically will remain silent to protect their parents. Making it safe for children to ask questions and express their preferences without the risk of alienating those they love most is extremely important. Providing honest answers also helps children feel trust in the people caring for them.

With the exception of emancipated minors, children younger than 18 years do not possess competency (the legal ability to make decisions for themselves); however, they can participate in decision making if they possess sufficient capacity (ie, ability to understand the risks, benefits, and alternatives as they relate to a specific decision). In general, at the developmental age of 14 years, children have the cognitive skills needed to have decision-making capacity, although this should be evaluated for each child and each decision. Children younger than 14 years who have lived with a chronic severe illness may have had enough experience in the healthcare setting to have developed insight beyond their chronological age into health-related issues. Although children younger than 18 years cannot provide consent for treatments, they can be involved in decision making and provide assent. Even when children do not have decision-making capacity, it is important to listen to them and take their wishes into consideration when setting goals of care. Children should be asked on a regular basis how they feel their treatments are going and if there is anything their parents or care team can help them achieve.

Children may want to document the things that are most important to them about their medical care. Although the advance directives filled out by adults typically are not appropriate for use with children, there are tools that have been specially designed to elicit children's goals and wishes. These tools include "My Wishes" and "Voicing My Choices."[38]

When exploring a child's goals, it can be helpful to be familiar with common goals of care for children at different developmental ages. Infants and preschool-aged children typically want the presence of loved ones as well as love and affection. They fear being separated from the people who are close to them. School-aged children often want to be with friends and return to school. Teenagers often will pull away from their parents to develop a sense of self and personal identity. They often realize that their ability to experience the benefits and responsibilities of adulthood may be limited, and they may want to experience new activities, graduate from high school, engage in sexual activity, get married, or live independently. Supporting these goals can be difficult for parents of sick children who want to keep their child close and not lose any of the precious time they have left with their child. The palliative care team can help parents understand their child's developmental needs and help teenagers express their wishes.

Like other things, decision-making skills improve with practice, age, and maturity. It is important to give children who are chronically ill the opportunity to develop decision-making skills. If this is not done, they may become overwhelmed as they get older and are asked to make their own medical decisions and set their own goals of care. As with adults, children typically want control over their experiences and are glad to be involved in decision making at a developmentally appropriate level. They have opinions about how and when therapies are provided and tests are done. Even very young children can be given simple choices about their care, such as which arm to have blood drawn from or whether to take medication as a pill or liquid. As children get older they should be involved in increasingly complex decisions. When there are two options, both of which are acceptable to the parents, the child should be involved in making the final decision.

It is not uncommon for parents to request that care providers not disclose information to a child about his or her illness. These situations must be navigated carefully following the steps described in **Table 10.5**. In particular, decisions about when to disclose to a child that he or she is dying can be difficult for families, but when parents make the decision to talk with their child about dying, they rarely regret the choice. In one study of 429 parents in Sweden who had lost their children to cancer, 147 reported having talked with their child about death (34%). None of these parents regretted having talked with their children. Of the remaining parents who did not speak with their children about death, 27% regretted their decision to forgo this conversation.[39]

Table 10.5 A Step-Wise Approach to Nondisclosure

Prevention: Engage in open dialogue from the start of the relationship.

Remain calm and respond empathically throughout.

Understand disclosure as a process, not a "tell-all" moment in time.

Determine cultural and religious context for information sharing and the hierarchy for decision making.

Try to understand the family's viewpoint: What are they afraid will happen?

Determine what the child already knows and has questions about.

Brainstorm possible solutions together with the family.

Ensure family information disclosure occurs in a step-wise fashion.

Engage the interdisciplinary team in information gathering and sharing.

Negotiate a solution: Reiterate honesty and fidelity to the child as your primary patient but respect a family-centered approach.

Create a mechanism for involved caregivers to discuss issues and concerns or to opt out of direct care.

If there is an impasse, enlist an outside advisor (eg, extended family, ethics consultant, family religious leader).

Adapted from Zieber S, Friebert S. Pediatric cancer care: special issues in ethical decision making. Cancer Treat Res. 2008;140 93-115; and Chaitin E, Rosielle D. Responding to requests for non-disclosure of medical information. Fast Facts and Concepts #219. Medical Colleges of Wisconsin End of Life/Palliative Care Resource Center website. www.eperc.mcw.edu/EPERC/ FastFactsIndex/ff_219.htm. Published September 2009. Reproduced from Carter BS, Levetown M, Friebert SE. Palliative Care for Infants, Children, and Adolescents: A Practical Handbook. 2nd ed. New York, NY: The Johns Hopkins University Press; 2011. © 2011 The Johns Hopkins University Press. Reprinted with permission.

Estimating and Communicating Prognosis

Determining the prognosis for children with serious illnesses can be very difficult because life-threatening diseases of childhood sometimes are rare, often have a variable course, and frequently are characterized by an unpredictable trajectory that often extends over many years and is marked by multiple life-threatening exacerbations. Although the discussion about prognosis may be difficult, when there is significant uncertainty about how a child's disease will progress, these conversations can be helpful to parents and give them a sense of control.[40,41]

There are few tools for estimating prognosis that are specific to children. As with adults, a child's functional status, signs, symptoms, physiologic variables, and specific disease all should be taken into account. In children with cancer, the Lansky Play Performance Scale (**Table 10.6**) can be used to assess functional status.[42]

Table 10.6 Lansky Play Performance Scale[42]

SCORE	DESCRIPTION
100	Fully active, normal
90	Minor restrictions in physically strenuous activity
80	Active, but tires more quickly
70	Both greater restriction of and less time spent in active play
60	Up and around, but minimal active play; keeps busy with quieter activities
50	Gets dressed, but lies around much of the day; no active play; able to participate in all quiet play and activities
40	Mostly in bed; participates in quiet activities
30	In bed; needs assistance even for quiet play
20	Often sleeping; play entirely limited to very passive activities
10	No play; does not get out of bed
0	Unresponsive

From Lansky SB, List MA, Lansky LL, Ritter-Sterr C, Miller DR. The measurement of performance in childhood cancer patients. Cancer. 1987;60(1):1651-1656. © 1987 John Wiley & Sons, Inc. Reprinted with permission.

The approach described in chapter 7 should be used when communicating with parents about their child's prognosis. The "caveat-ball-park-exception" format can be very useful for conveying prognosis in the setting of significant uncertainty.

Self-Care and Care of Team

The concepts of countertransference, burnout, and self-care, which are discussed in section 6D (p. 132), are essential for providers to understand and address so they can provide compassionate, self-aware care to children and their families. In addition, providers may be at risk for developing compassion fatigue, which can result from caring for others with emotional pain.[43] Compassion fatigue has some similar characteristics to posttraumatic stress disorder, except it is a response to witnessing the emotional stress of another person instead of one's own trauma.[44] It is different from burnout in that it develops from the relationship between the clinician and patient, whereas burnout develops from stressful interaction with the work environment. Symptoms of compassion fatigue include hyperarousal (irritability, outbursts of anger, disturbed sleep, and hypervigilance), avoidance (avoiding thoughts, feelings, and conversations associated with a patient's suffering), and re-experiencing (having intrusive thoughts or dreams and distress in response to reminders of bearing witness to the suffering of another).[43,44]

Although some providers experience compassion fatigue, other providers feel rewarded by their work with very sick and dying children. They may experience satisfaction when a death is peaceful or when a family finds meaning in their child's life. They may gain perspective on what is most important to them in life, contemplate their own mortality, and experience personal growth.[43]

One of the best ways to avoid compassion fatigue and foster the capacity for growth and personal satisfaction is to develop self-awareness.[43] Mindfulness meditation,[45] reflective writing,[46,47] and participation in peer support groups[48,49] can all enhance self-awareness.

As well as caring for themselves, it is important for providers to be aware of the emotional reactions of other individuals who are involved in the care of a sick child. Pediatric palliative care providers are often in the position of needing to acknowledge and address the strong emotional reactions other providers have when caring for a very sick or dying child. Allowing team members to express emotions and concerns can improve team function and cohesion. Support may be provided to distressed clinicians through one-on-one conversations, group debriefs, and education that raises awareness of burnout, compassion fatigue, and ways to prevent and address these conditions.

10H | Last-Resort Options

Proportionate Palliative Sedation

Proportionate palliative sedation can be used when an imminently dying child is experiencing intractable physical symptoms that do not respond to other therapies (**Table 10.7**). The framework for considering proportionate palliative sedation and the guidelines for initiating it provided in section 8A (p. 173) should be applied. Although the same medications are used for both children and adults, the medication dosing is different. The first-line therapy is treatment with a benzodiazepine unless the patient has received significant doses of these medications in the past. In this case, the child may have developed a tolerance to benzodiazepines that makes the medications ineffective in achieving the level of sedation needed to relieve the child's symptoms. Phenobarbital is a second-line therapy.

Table 10.7 Medications for Palliative Sedation in Children

NB: Opioids used to treat pain or dyspnea should be continued in this process.

MEDICATION	DOSAGE	COMMENT
Midazolam	Bolus: 0.05 mg/kg IV push over 2 minutes. Repeat dose every 10 minutes until patient is comfortable or a predetermined max dose is reached Maintenance: 0.02 mg/kg/hour or an hourly rate of 25% of the loading dose needed to achieve patient comfort Routes: IV or SC	Medication most often used for palliative sedation Young patients may require higher mg/kg doses
Lorazepam	Bolus: 0.05 mg/kg Maintenance: 0.01 mg/kg/hour-0.1 mg/kg/hour Routes: PO, SC, IV, buccal	When given IV, may repeat the dose after 10 minutes
Phenobarbital	Bolus: 3 mg/kg-5mg/kg slow IV injection repeated every 10-15 minutes until comfortable to a max. of 30 mg/kg Maintenance: Neonates: 3 mg/kg/24 hours-5 mg/kg/24 hours divided twice a day Infants: 5 mg/kg/24 hours-6 mg/kg/24 hours divided twice a day 1-5 year old: 6 mg/kg/24 hours-8 mg/kg/24 hours divided twice a day 6-12 year old: 4 mg/kg/24 hours-6 mg/kg/24 hours divided twice a day >12 year old: 1 mg/kg/24 hours-3 mg/kg/24 hours divided twice a day Routes: see comments	Long acting Loading dose may be given IM, IV, or PR When administering IM, dose may need to be divided and given into more than one site When administering loading dose IV, give 1 mg/kg/minute to a max. of 30 mg/minute Maintenance dose may be given intermittently IV, IM, PR, or by NG/NJ/G tube Maintenance dose can be given by continuous infusion IV or SC

G, gastric; IM, intramuscular; IV, intravenous; NG, nasogastric; NJ, nasojejunal; PO, oral; PR, rectal; SC, subcutaneous.

Ventilator Withdrawal

The preparation for ventilator withdrawal in children and adults is the same (see section 8B [p. 177]). Pediatric providers should be particularly sensitive when assessing the emotional and spiritual needs of the family prior to the ventilator withdrawal. Attention should be given to creating a comfortable space in which to perform the procedure. Because infants and children are frequently smaller and more portable than adults, some special wishes of the family, such as withdrawing the ventilator in a specific location (eg, outdoors), may be more easily accommodated. Providers should assess the family's wishes in terms of how they would like to spend the time immediately prior to and after the ventilator withdrawal. There may be rituals, spiritual practices, or special goodbyes that the family would like to plan. Providers should also make sure that the family has the opportunity to do memory-making activities such as making hand- and footprints or taking photographs prior to the withdrawal. Depending on the size of the child, it may be possible to allow a parent to hold the child in his or her arms during the procedure, and this should be offered when appropriate. If holding the child is not possible, parents may choose to lie in bed with the child to provide more intimacy. Providing more space or a larger bed may be necessary in these situations.

Once the family's needs have been assessed and there is a plan for the time immediately preceding and following the withdrawal of the ventilator, the care team should meet to ensure that everyone is aware of the family's wishes and that there is a step-by-step plan in place. During this meeting, the role of each team member can be defined, plans for medication doses and delivery can be discussed, and the setup of the space can be reviewed.

In most cases, there is some uncertainty about how long the child will live after the ventilator is withdrawn. The family should be prepared for the child to die shortly after the ventilator is withdrawn or to live for hours or even days after the procedure. If the family is expecting the child to die immediately after the ventilator is withdrawn but the child instead lives for many hours or days, the family may question the expertise of the medical team and may experience added emotional distress.

As described in section 8B (p. 177), both immediate extubation or terminal wean are appropriate approaches to ventilator withdrawal in children, but generally immediate extubation is preferred. Opioids and benzodiazepines are the primary medications used to provide comfort in the setting of ventilator withdrawal. Consideration also should be given to secretion management. IV fluids, total parenteral nutrition, and tube feeds should be stopped at least 12 hours prior to the withdrawal of the ventilator, when possible. These therapies can cause increased secretions, leading to respiratory distress at the time of ventilator withdrawal. An anticholinergic medication, such as glycopyrrolate, should be available for use as needed prior to or after the procedure. If there is any risk of bleeding from the lungs after extubation, leaving the endotracheal tube in place and simply disconnecting the child from the ventilator should be considered. Bleeding at the time of extubation is very traumatic for both the family and care team.

- For patients who have not been on opioids or benzodiazepines, shortly before withdrawal give a 0.1-mg/kg to 0.2-mg/kg (for infants 6 months and younger, give 0.03 mg/kg to 0.06 mg/kg) IV bolus of morphine or equivalent, followed by an infusion of 0.02 mg/kg/hour to 0.05 mg/kg/hour IV (for infants 6 months and younger, give 0.006 mg/kg/hour to 0.015 mg/kg/hour IV), as well as a 0.05 mg/kg to 0.1 mg/kg IV bolus of midazolam followed by an infusion at any hourly rate of 25% of the bolus dose needed to achieve comfort.
- If the patient is already on continuous opioids, give a bolus of two times the current hourly rate and increase the hourly infusion rate by 30%.
- If distress ensues after ventilator withdrawal, aggressive and immediate symptom control is imperative. Use morphine, 0.1 mg/kg to 0.2 mg/kg (for infants 6 months and younger, give 0.03 mg/kg to 0.06 mg/kg) IV bolus every 10 minutes or use a bolus dose that is two times the hourly rate, and midazolam, 0.05 mg/kg to 0.1 mg/kg IV every 10 minutes prn. Once the patient is comfortable, increase the

infusion rates by 30% or more based on the amount of medication that was required to achieve comfort.

- Specific dosages are less important than achieving symptom relief; a general goal is to eliminate signs of respiratory distress, such as grimacing and agitation.

10I | Care During the Last Hours of Life
What to Prepare For

Section 9A (p. 191) describes the symptoms that patients may experience in their last hours and days of life. Dying children experience the same changes at the end of life as adults. Whether a child is being cared for in the hospital, a long-term care facility, or at home, it is important to anticipate common end-of-life symptoms and ensure that appropriate medication orders and equipment are available. Typically, it is important to have orders for opioids for pain or dyspnea, benzodiazepines for agitation or seizures, anticholinergics for secretions, and an appropriate medication for nausea. Dosing for medications commonly used in pediatric palliative care is available in Table 10.3. Close attention should be paid to the medication concentration and route of delivery. At the end of life, medications often are given buccally. If this route is used, medications should be sufficiently concentrated so the volume is not too large for the child. Patients' equipment needs will differ depending on their age, diagnosis, and symptoms, but equipment to consider includes a hospital bed, bedside table, oxygen, suction, and bedside commode.

Before death is imminent, it is helpful to discuss with the family their preferences for the child's location of death. This is often done within the context of goals of care. The parents should be given a full range of choices and be allowed to explore the benefits and burdens of different care settings at the end of life. Available choices will depend on the resources in the child's community, but they might include a hospital general medical unit or oncology unit, an intensive care unit, a long-term care facility, an inpatient hospice facility, or the family's home. Whenever possible, the parents' preferences should be honored. The parents also should understand that they are always able to change their mind about the most appropriate care setting based on the needs of their child. One study of pediatric oncology patients found that planning a location of death was associated with more deaths at home and fewer hospital admissions. Parents who planned for the location of their child's death were more likely to feel prepared for the end of life, be very comfortable with the location in which the death occurred, and be less likely to have preferred a different location of death.[50]

Consideration also should be given as to whether an autopsy should be offered. Many children who are cared for by palliative care providers have rare or undiagnosed conditions. An autopsy may help the family by providing additional information about the cause of the patient's condition. The information obtained through an autopsy also may be helpful if parents are considering having more children. Parents should be aware that limited autopsies including only specific organs can be performed. DNA banking is available if a diagnosis cannot be made and the family would like the option to conduct further genetic testing as advances are made in the ability to diagnose rare conditions.

After the death of a child, it is important to give the family sufficient space and time to say goodbye and to respect religious rituals and practices. It can be very difficult for parents and other family members to part from the body of a child. In some cases, it may be helpful to allow family members to bathe and dress the child after the death. If the family wants to keep the child in the home setting for a period of days, dry ice can be used to preserve the body. When the family does leave the child's body, it is important that they feel the body will be well cared for. In the hospital setting, there may be policies about preparing a body before it is sent to the morgue that require actions such as removing the child's clothing or tying the hands together. If these polices exist, it is best to allow the family to say goodbye before preparing the body for the morgue. In the home or inpatient hospice setting, it is helpful to prepare the mortuary for receiving the body of a child. If the child is small enough, it may be comforting to allow the parents to carry the body and place it in the arms of the mortician instead of watching it being placed on a gurney and covered. Parents and other family members will carry their last memories of the child with them forever. It is important to make these memories as peaceful and comforting as possible.

Grief and Bereavement

A child's death causes distress throughout the entire family system. Because the grief process starts at the time of the child's diagnosis, it is important that the family has access to grief support both during the child's illness and after his or her death. A parent's grief after the loss of a child can be intense and long lasting.[51] One study found higher rates of anxiety and depression in bereaved parents compared with the general population 4 to 6 years after a child's death.[52] Although families never "get over" the loss of a child, they can learn to integrate memories of their child into a healthy family life. Two factors that make parents more likely to work through their grief are sharing their problems with others during the child's illness and access to psychological support during the last months of the child's life.[53] Although it can be normal for the grief process to continue long after the loss of a child, when parents or other family members experience intense grieving over an extended period of time that causes significant disruptions in their social or work lives, they may be experiencing complicated grief that will require treatment. The differences between normal grief and complicated grief are reviewed in section 9B (p. 200).

The two parents of a child who has died often grieve differently, both in style and timing. These differences can cause significant strain in their relationship. Providers can help parents understand the differences in the way people grieve to decrease the tension that may occur in the parents' relationship after the child's death. It can be explained that grievers may be intuitive, instrumental, or blended in their grief style.[54] Intuitive grievers experience feelings intensely and express these feelings outwardly. Experiencing and expressing feelings is an important part of moving through grief for this group of individuals. Instrumental grievers experience feelings less intensely and use thinking to move through their grief. They may be reluctant to talk about their feelings, instead using problem-solving strategies to attempt to master their emotions. Blended grievers integrate components of both patterns. It may be difficult for parents with different grieving styles to understand how the other is processing their grief, especially if one partner needs quiet time to think and the other needs to be able to talk and express emotion. These differences can cause misunderstandings, anger, guilt, loneliness, and resentment. An understanding that there are different styles of grieving and that it is important to recognize and support each other's grief styles can help decrease the strain.

It is also important to prepare families for the possibility of renewed feelings of intense grief on occasions that would have been important benchmarks in their child's life, such as birthdays, graduations, or holidays. They should be reassured that these exacerbations of grief do not represent mental illness or emotional instability.

Particular care should be given to attending to the grief of siblings and other children in the family. Siblings must negotiate both their own grief and the distance they may feel between themselves and their parents, who are immersed in their own grieving process. It is normal for children to alternate between expressing their grief and seemingly ignoring the situation. Parents should be warned that children often use play as a coping mechanism. Playing or seemingly ignoring the situation for periods of time does not mean that the child is indifferent or does not care.

Parents often try to protect siblings by limiting their involvement in the medical care of their sick sibling, particularly at the end of life. This can cause siblings to feel abandoned and excluded. Most siblings desire open and honest communication within the family, adequate information from clinicians, involvement in the care of the sick sibling, and support to continue their own interests and activities.[55,56] Keeping to routines can enhance children's feelings of safety and comfort, and continuing to set limits and enforce discipline can help them understand that they are still important. Children's school performance may decline during a period of grieving, and they may act out or withdraw. It is particularly important to be aware that many children experience guilt after the loss of a sibling, but unrelenting guilt may require psychological intervention.

Further Discussion

1. What are three ways in which palliative care programs can support children and their parents?

2. How does the "Concurrent Care for Children Requirement" included in the Affordable Care Act affect access to hospice care? What population of children can benefit from the requirement?

3. At what developmental age are children able to use pain assessment tools to rate the severity of their pain? What tools are most appropriate for use in young children? At what developmental age are children able to use visual analog scales and 0-to-10 verbal numeric scales to rate their pain?

4. When prescribing opioids to children who are 6 months of age or younger, how should the opioid dose be adjusted? Why is this dose adjustment necessary?

5. What adjustment should be made when switching from glycopyrrolate administered orally or via gastric tube to glycopyrrolate administered parenterally?

6. What are three potential benefits of placing a gastric tube in a neurologically impaired child? What are three potential burdens?

7. What are two differences between the evaluation of delirium in adults and young children?

8. What are three ways in which children can create a legacy that expresses their values?

9. What are common goals of care for children at the following developmental ages?

   - Infants and preschool children
   - School-aged children
   - Teenagers

continued

Further Discussion *continued*

10. What is compassion fatigue and how is it different from burnout? Name three ways in which compassion fatigue can be avoided.

11. List three benefits that can result from discussions with parents about the preferred location for their child's death.

12. List and describe three different styles of grieving. How can differences in styles of grieving affect the relationship between two grieving parents?

References

1. Himelstein BP, Hilden JM, Boldt AM, Weissman D. Pediatric palliative care. *N Engl J Med.* 2004;350(17):1752-1762.

2. Concurrent Care for Children Implementation Toolkit; Section 2302 of the Patient Protection and Affordable Care Act. www.nhpco.org/sites/default/files/public/ChiPPS/CCCR_Toolkit.pdf. Accessed September 2, 2013.

3. Bluebond-Langner M, Belasco JB, DeMesquita Wander M. "I want to live, until I don't want to live anymore": involving children with life-threatening and life-shortening illnesses in decision making about care and treatment. *Nurs Clin North Am.* 2010;45(3):329-343.

4. van Breemen C. Using play therapy in paediatric palliative care: listening to the story and caring for the body. *Int J Palliat Nurs.* 2009;15(10):510-514.

5. Knapp C, Madden V, Wang H, Curtis C, Sloyer P, Shenkman E. Music therapy in an integrated pediatric palliative care program. *Am J Hosp Palliat Care.* 2009;26(6):449-455.

6. Kool R, Lawver T. Play therapy: considerations and applications for the practitioner. *Psychiatry.* 2010;7(10):19-24.

7. Geue K, Goetze H, Buttstaedt M, Kleinert E, Richter D, Singer S. An overview of art therapy interventions for cancer patients and the results of research. *Complement Ther Med.* 2010;18(3-4):160-170.

8. Bailey B, Daoust R, Doyon-Trottier E, Dauphin-Pierre S, Gravel J. Validation and properties of the verbal numeric scale in children with acute pain. *Pain.* 2010;149(2):216-221.

9. Shields BJ, Cohen DM, Harbeck-Weber C, Powers JD, Smith GA. Pediatric pain measurement using a visual analogue scale: a comparison of two teaching methods. *Clin Pediatrics.* 2003;42(3):227-234.

10. Manworren RC, Hynan LS. Clinical validation of FLACC: preverbal patient pain scale. *Pediatric Nurs.* 2003;29(2):140-146.

11. Krechel SW, Bildner J. CRIES: a new neonatal postoperative pain measurement score. Initial testing of validity and reliability. *Paediatric Anaesth.* 1995;5(1):53-61.

12. Merkel SI, Voepel-Lewis T, Shayevitz JR, Malviya S. The FLACC: a behavioral scale for scoring postoperative pain in young children. *Pediatric Nurs.* 1997;23(3):293-297.

13. Friedrichsdorf SJ, Nugent AP, Strobl AQ. Codeine-associated pediatric deaths despite using recommended dosing guidelines: three case reports. *J Opioid Manage.* 2013;9(2):151-155.

14. Voelker R. Children's deaths linked with postsurgical codeine. *JAMA.* 2012;308(10):963.

15. Williams DG, Patel A, Howard RF. Pharmacogenetics of codeine metabolism in an urban population of children and its implications for analgesic reliability. *Brit J Anaesth.* 2002;89(6):839-845.

16. Berde CB, Sethna NF. Analgesics for the treatment of pain in children. *N Engl J Med.* 2002;347(14):1094-1103.

17. Khan FI, Reddy RC, Baptist AP. Pediatric Dyspnea Scale for use in hospitalized patients with asthma. *J Allergy Clin Immunol.* 2009;123(3):660-664.

18. McGrath PJ, Pianosi PT, Unruh AM, Buckley CP. Dalhousie dyspnea scales: construct and content validity of pictorial scales for measuring dyspnea. *BMC Pediatrics.* 2005;5:33.

19. Feudtner C, Kang TI, Hexem KR, et al. Pediatric palliative care patients: a prospective multicenter cohort study. *Pediatrics.* 2011;127(6):1094-1101.

20. Naureckas SM, Christoffel KK. Nasogastric or gastrostomy feedings in children with neurologic disabilities. *Clin Ped.* 1994;33(6):353-359.

21. Sullivan PB, Juszczak E, Bachlet AM, et al. Impact of gastrostomy tube feeding on the quality of life of carers of children with cerebral palsy. *Dev Med Child Neurol.* 2004;46(12):796-800.

22. Bateman DN, Rawlins MD, Simpson JM. Extrapyramidal reactions with metoclopramide. *Brit Med J.* 1985;291(6500):930-932.

23. Vickers AJ. Can acupuncture have specific effects on health? A systematic review of acupuncture antiemesis trials. *J Royal Soc Med.* 1996;89(6):303-311.

24. Pashankar DS, Bishop WP. Efficacy and optimal dose of daily polyethylene glycol 3350 for treatment of constipation and encopresis in children. *J Pediatrics.* 2001;139(3):428-432.

25. March JS, Silva S, Petrycki S, et al. The Treatment for Adolescents with Depression Study (TADS): long-term effectiveness and safety outcomes. *Arch Gen Psychiatry.* 2007;64(10):1132-1143.

26. Kanitz JL, Camus ME, Seifert G. Keeping the balance—an overview of mind-body therapies in pediatric oncology. *Complement Ther Med.* 2013;21 Suppl 1:S20-25.

27. Halm MA. The healing power of the human-animal connection. *Am J Crit Care.* 2008;17(4):373-376.

28. Gothelf D, Rubinstein M, Shemesh E, et al. Pilot study: fluvoxamine treatment for depression and anxiety disorders in children and adolescents with cancer. *J Am Acad Child Adolesc Psychiatry.* 2005;44(12):1258-1262.

29. DeJong M, Fombonne E. Citalopram to treat depression in pediatric oncology. *J Child Adolesc Psychopharmacol.* 2007;17(3):371-377.

30. Pfefferbaum-Levine B, Kumor K, Cangir A, Choroszy M, Roseberry EA. Tricyclic antidepressants for children with cancer. *Am J Psychiatry.* 1983;140(8):1074-1076.

31. Maisami M, Sohmer BH, Coyle JT. Combined use of tricyclic antidepressants and neuroleptics in the management of terminally ill children: a report on three cases. *J Am Acad Child Psychiatry.* 1985;24(4):487-489.

32. Walling VR, Pfefferbaum B. The use of methylphenidate in a depressed adolescent with AIDS. *J Dev Behav Pediatr.* 1990;11(4):195-197.

33. Turkel SB, Tavare CJ. Delirium in children and adolescents. *J Neuropsychiatry Clin Neurosci.* 2003;15(4):431-435.

34. Schieveld JN, Leroy PL, van Os J, Nicolai J, Vos GD, Leentjens AF. Pediatric delirium in critical illness: phenomenology, clinical correlates and treatment response in 40 cases in the pediatric intensive care unit. *Intensive Care Med.* 2007;33(6):1033-1040.

35. Wolfe J, Grier HE, Klar N, et al. Symptoms and suffering at the end of life in children with cancer. *N Engl J Med.* 2000;342(5):326-333.

36. Yee JD, Berde CB. Dextroamphetamine or methylphenidate as adjuvants to opioid analgesia for adolescents with cancer. *J Pain Symptom Manage.* 1994;9(2):122-125.

37. Sood A, Barton DL, Loprinzi CL. Use of methylphenidate in patients with cancer. *Am J Hosp Palliat Care.* 2006;23(1):35-40.

38. Wiener L, Zadeh S, Battles H, et al. Allowing adolescents and young adults to plan their end-of-life care. *Pediatrics.* 2012;130(5):897-905.

39. Kreicbergs U, Valdimarsdottir U, Onelov E, Henter JI, Steineck G. Talking about death with children who have severe malignant disease. *N Engl J Med.* 2004;351(12):1175-1186.

40. Mack JW, Cook EF, Wolfe J, Grier HE, Cleary PD, Weeks JC. Understanding of prognosis among parents of children with cancer: parental optimism and the parent-physician interaction. *J Clin Oncol.* 2007;25(11):1357-1362.

41. Mack JW, Wolfe J, Grier HE, Cleary PD, Weeks JC. Communication about prognosis between parents and physicians of children with cancer: parent preferences and the impact of prognostic information. *J Clin Oncol.* 2006;24(33):5265-5270.

42. Lansky SB, List MA, Lansky LL, Ritter-Sterr C, Miller DR. The measurement of performance in childhood cancer patients. *Cancer.* 1987;60(7):1651-1656.

43. Kearney MK, Weininger RB, Vachon ML, Harrison RL, Mount BM. Self-care of physicians caring for patients at the end of life: "Being connected... a key to my survival." *JAMA.* 2009;301(11):1155-1164.

44. Figley CR. In: Figley CR, ed. *Compassion Fatigue: Coping with Secondary Traumatic Stress Disorder in Those Who treat the Traumatized.* London: Brunner-Routledge; 1995.

45. Epstein RM. Mindful practice. *JAMA.* 1999;282(9):833-839.

46. Frisina PG, Borod JC, Lepore SJ. A meta-analysis of the effects of written emotional disclosure on the health outcomes of clinical populations. *J Nerv Ment Dis.* 2004;192(9):629-634.

47. Harris AH. Does expressive writing reduce health care utilization? A meta-analysis of randomized trials. *J Consult Clin Psychol.* 2006;74(2):243-252.

48. Rabinowitz S, Kushnir T, Ribak J. Preventing burnout: increasing professional self efficacy in primary care nurses in a Balint Group. *AAOHN.* 1996;44(1):28-32.

49. Kjeldmand D, Holmstrom I, Rosenqvist U. Balint training makes GPs thrive better in their job. *Patient Educ Couns.* 2004;55(2):230-235.

50. Dussel V, Kreicbergs U, Hilden JM, et al. Looking beyond where children die: determinants and effects of planning a child's location of death. *J Pain Symptom Manage.* 2009;37(1):33-43.

51. Whittam EH. Terminal care of the dying child. Psychosocial implications of care. *Cancer.* 1993;71(10 Suppl):3450-3462.

52. Kreicbergs U, Valdimarsdottir U, Onelov E, Henter JI, Steineck G. Anxiety and depression in parents 4-9 years after the loss of a child owing to a malignancy: a population-based follow-up. *Psychol Med.* 2004;34(8):1431-1441.

53. Kreicbergs UC, Lannen P, Onelov E, Wolfe J. Parental grief after losing a child to cancer: impact of professional and social support on long-term outcomes. *J Clin Oncol.* 2007;25(22):3307-3312.

54. Martin TL, Doka KJ. *Men Don't Cry...Women Do: Transcending Gender Stereotypes of Grief.* Philadelphia, PA: Brunner/Mazel; 2000.

55. Wilkins KL, Woodgate RL. A review of qualitative research on the childhood cancer experience from the perspective of siblings: a need to give them a voice. *J Pediatr Oncol Nurs.* 2005;22(6):305-319.

56. Nolbris M, Hellstrom AL. Siblings' needs and issues when a brother or sister dies of cancer. *J Pediatr Oncol Nurs.* 2005;22(4):227-233.

Appendix

Web Resources

American Academy of Hospice and Palliative Medicine (AAHPM)
aahpm.org, aahpmblog.com
AAHPM is the professional organization of physicians dedicated to excellence in palliative care. This site lists information about publications, meetings, and many other resources.

Caring Connections
www.caringinfo.org
This program of the National Hospice and Palliative Care Organization is a national consumer engagement initiative aimed at improving care at the end of life. Advance directives for every state can be downloaded for free.

Center to Advance Palliative Care (CAPC)
www.capc.org
CAPC provides healthcare professionals with the tools, training, and technical assistance necessary to start and sustain successful palliative care programs in hospitals and other healthcare settings.

Compassion and Choices
www.compassionandchoices.org
Compassion and Choices provides service, education, and advocacy for improved care and expanded options at the end of life.

Education in Palliative and End-of-Life Care (EPEC)
www.epec.net
EPEC combines didactic sessions, videotape presentations, interactive discussions, and practical exercises to educate all healthcare professionals on the essential clinical competencies in palliative care.

End of Life/Palliative Education Resource Center (EPERC)

www.eperc.mcw.edu

EPERC shares educational resource material with the community of health professional educators involved in palliative care education. EPERC offers starter kits and group educational offerings for hospice medical directors, medical students, and those preparing for board certification.

Hospice and Palliative Medicine SmartBriefs

https://www2.smartbrief.com/getSample.jsp?b=AAHPM

This digital news service provides "must read" industry news gleaned from thousands of sources and summarized twice weekly.

Hospice and Palliative Nurses Association (HPNA)

www.hpna.org

HPNA is the nation's largest and oldest professional nursing organization dedicated to promoting excellence in hospice and palliative care.

International Association for Hospice and Palliative Care (IAHPC)

www.hospicecare.com

IAHPC promotes communication and facilitates and provides education by being an information resource for patients, professionals, healthcare providers, and policy makers around the world. The website hosts an extensive bookstore, evaluation tools, review articles, and more.

The National Consensus Project (NCP) for Quality Palliative Care

www.nationalconsensusproject.org

The NCP represents a coalition of leading palliative care organizations that developed *Clinical Practice Guidelines for Quality Palliative Care* as a national consensus of what the standard of palliative care should be.

National Hospice and Palliative Care Organization (NHPCO)

www.nhpco.org

NHPCO represents hospice and palliative care programs and professionals in the United States. The website allows users to find hospice providers. Members can access many documents, particularly around regulatory and administrative aspects of hospice care.

National Palliative Care Research Center (NPCRC)

www.npcrc.org

NPCRC is committed to stimulating, developing, and funding research directed at improving care for seriously ill patients and their families. Its collections of measurement tools and funding sources are particularly valuable.

National Quality Forum: A National Framework and Preferred Practices for Palliative and Hospice Care Quality

www.qualityforum.org/Publications/2006/12/A_National_Framework_ and_Preferred_Practices_for_Palliative_and_Hospice_Care_Quality.aspx

This site offers a comprehensive framework for evaluating the quality of palliative and hospice care, a set of 38 preferred practices for delivering high-quality palliative and hospice care, and 9 recommendations for research to improve upon the measurement and evaluation of palliative and hospice care.

PalliativeDoctors

PalliativeDoctors.org

This patient- and family-focused website was developed by AAHPM and is designed to serve as a resource about palliative care and hospice.

Pallimed

www.pallimed.org

Pallimed is an educational hospice and palliative medicine blog maintained by physicians in the field.

Social Work in Hospice and Palliative Care Network (SWHPN)

http://swhpn.org

SWHPN is a network of social work organizations and leaders who seek to advance the role of social work in hospice and palliative care.

Palliative Care Journals

American Journal of Hospice and Palliative Medicine
http://ajh.sagepub.com
This peer-reviewed journal provides an essential forum for articles covering all aspects of hospice and palliation from the medical and pharmaceutical to the administrative and social.

European Journal of Palliative Care (EJPC)
www.ejpc.eu.com
The official journal of the European Association for Palliative Care, *EJPC* aims to provide information for all professionals involved in the provision of palliative care by covering all aspects of the care of patients suffering from advanced, incurable disease.

Journal of Pain and Symptom Management (JPSM)
www.jpsmjournal.com
This international, peer-reviewed journal is the official journal of AAHPM, the US Cancer Pain Relief Committee, and NHPCO. *JPSM* publishes original articles describing qualitative and quantitative research.

Journal of Palliative Care
www.criugm.qc.ca/journalofpalliativecare
This journal, published by the Centre for Bioethics, is a Canadian-based, peer-reviewed, international, and interdisciplinary forum for practical, critical thought on palliative care and palliative medicine.

Journal of Palliative Medicine
www.liebertpub.com/JPM
This monthly interdisciplinary publication reports on the clinical, educational, legal, and ethical aspects of caring for seriously ill and dying patients.

Journal of Supportive Oncology

www.oncologypractice.com/supportiveoncology
This journal publishes review articles and original research relating to practical management issues in the palliative and supportive care of patients with neoplastic diseases.

Pain

www.journals.elsevier.com/pain
The official publication of the International Association for the Study of Pain, *Pain* publishes original research on the nature, mechanisms, and treatment of pain.

Palliative Medicine

pmj.sagepub.com
This journal is the multiprofessional journal of the European Association for Palliative Care.

Progress in Palliative Care

www.maneypublishing.com/index.php/journals/ppc
This journal is a multidisciplinary journal with an international perspective. It provides a major listing of the international research literature, including that which is novel and pertinent though not widely available.

Supportive Care in Cancer

www.link.springer.com/journal/520
This is the official journal of the Multinational Association of Supportive Care in Cancer, which aims to provide the most recent scientific and social information on all aspects of supportive care in cancer patients.

Index

A

abandonment, integrity and, 186
acetaminophen
    pain management, 17, 36t
    pediatric use of, 217, 218t
acupuncture, 78
acute pain crises
    description of, 29–30
    pediatric, 215
addiction
    characteristics of, 33
    opioid side effects, 32–34
    pediatric, 217
    risk factors, 32
adjustment disorder with anxious mood, 103
adjuvant analgesia, 34–35, 36t–38t, 217–223
adverse effects
    intolerable side effects, 32
    metoclopramide, 228
    secondary fatigue and, 113t
affective domain, 151t
age/aging, analgesic choices and, 18
agitation
    dying patients, 196
    management of, 192
    sedation agitation scale, 177t
AIDS, illness trajectories, 4
airway obstruction, malignant central, 49t
alendronate, 62
alprazolam, 109t
amantadine, for fatigue, 115, 115t
amiodarone, drug interactions, 27
amitriptyline
    for major depression, 108t
    pediatric use of, 221t
analgesics
    adjuvant agents, 34–35, 36t–38t, 217–223
    choice of, 17–18
    nonopioid, 17
    opioid, 13

anemia
    dyspnea and, 49t
    secondary fatigue and, 113t
anger, depression and, 101
angular stomatitis, 61
anorexia, secondary fatigue and, 113t
anorexia-cachexia syndrome, 159
anticholinergics
    dry mouth and, 62
    pain management, 38t
    secretion control and, 56
anticipatory grief, 200
anticonvulsants, pain management, 37t
antipsychotic agents, 98
antiretroviral agents, 27
anxiety
    assessment of, 101–103
    causes of, 104t
    in children, 232–233
    counseling for, 105–106
    dyspnea and, 48t
    management of, 192
    nausea, vomiting and, 76t
    serious illness and, 100
    treatment, 103–110, 109t–110t
anxiolytic therapy
    opioid toxicity and, 52
    opioids with, 50
    ventilator withdrawal and, 180
appetite, megestrol acetate and, 114
aprepitant, 77
aripiprazole, for delirium, 98
aromatherapy, for fatigue, 116
arrhythmias, methadone and, 26–27
art therapy, 232
artificial nutrition and hydration (ANH), 66–72
    education about, 70–71
    pediatric patients, 227–228
as-needed (prn) medication, 18
    calculations, 22
    dosage calculations, 21
    methadone, 28
    morphine, 28–29
ascites, dyspnea and, 49t
atropine
    for oral secretions, 57t